HANDBOOK OF
DYNAMIC
PSYCHOTHERAPY
FOR HIGHER LEVEL
PERSONALITY
PATHOLOGY

HANDBOOK OF
DYNAMIC
PSYCHOTHERAPY
FOR HIGHER LEVEL
PERSONALITY
PATHOLOGY

Eve Caligor, M.D.
Otto F. Kernberg, M.D.
John F. Clarkin, Ph.D.

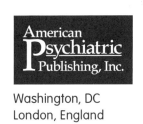

American Psychiatric Publishing, Inc.

Washington, DC
London, England

To purchase 25 to 99 copies of this or any other APPI title at a 20% discount, please contact APPI Customer Service at appi@psych.org or 800-368-5777. To purchase 100 or more copies of the same title, please e-mail us at bulksales@psych.org for a price quote.

Copyright © 2007 American Psychiatric Publishing, Inc.
ALL RIGHTS RESERVED

Manufactured in the United States of America on acid-free paper
11   10   09   08   07   5   4   3   2   1
First Edition

Typeset in Adobe's Janson Text, Univers, and VAG Rounded.

American Psychiatric Publishing, Inc.
1000 Wilson Boulevard
Arlington, VA 22209-3901
www.appi.org

Library of Congress Cataloging-in-Publication Data
Caligor, Eve, 1956–
  Handbook of dynamic psychotherapy for higher level personality pathology /
Eve Caligor, Otto F. Kernberg, John F. Clarkin. — 1st ed.
      p. ; cm.
  Includes bibliographical references and index.
  ISBN 978-1-58562-212-2 (hbk. : alk. paper)
 1. Psychodynamic psychotherapy. 2. Personality disorders—Treatment.
I. Kernberg, Otto F., 1928– II. Clarkin, John F. III. Title.
  [DNLM: 1. Personality Disorders—therapy. 2. Psychotherapy—methods.
WM 190 C153h 2007]

  RC489.P72C35 2007
  616.89'14--dc22

                                                                2006036112

British Library Cataloguing in Publication Data
A CIP record is available from the British Library.

CONTENTS

PART I
Theoretical Understanding of
Higher Level Personality Pathology

PART II
Psychotherapeutic Treatment of
Higher Level Personality Pathology

PART III

Patient Assessment, Phases of Treatment, and Combining DPHP With Other Treatments

PREFACE

This book describes a specific form of psychodynamic treatment for personality pathology, which we have called *dynamic psychotherapy for higher level personality pathology* (DPHP). The treatment is based on contemporary psychodynamic object relations theory, which focuses on the ways in which an individual's psychological life is organized around internalized relationship patterns, referred to as *internal object relations.* In this treatment, we explore and ultimately modify the patient's internalized relationship patterns as they are played out in his current relationships. For readers who are relatively unfamiliar with object relations theory, we devote the first three chapters of this handbook to introducing the theory underlying this treatment.

The model of treatment described in this handbook is an outgrowth of *transference-focused psychotherapy* (TFP). TFP is a psychodynamic treatment for borderline personality, which has been developed and empirically tested at the Personality Disorders Institute of the Sanford Weill Cornell Medical College. TFP is unusual among long-term psychodynamic treatments in that 1) it was developed to treat a specific form of psychopathology, 2) the techniques of TFP are clearly described in a treatment manual, and 3) TFP has been empirically studied.

While teaching TFP at the Columbia University Center for Psychoanalytic Training and Research, we were struck by the absence of a treatment comparable to TFP for higher level personality pathology. This volume is intended to fill that gap and to serve as a companion volume to the TFP manual. Together, this handbook and the TFP manual provide a comprehensive description of an object-relations theory based approach to treatment of patients with personality disorders, embedded in an integrated model of personality.

This handbook is written for students of psychotherapy as well as for experienced clinicians. While we describe the treatment as clearly and specifically as possible, there is no question that a book of this kind must be somewhat sophisticated if it is to be useful. For the benefit of those first learning dynamic psychotherapy, we clearly and specifically explain the underlying theory, as well as the basic elements of DPHP. By describing goals, strategies, and tactics of DPHP, we help the reader to appreciate the rationale for the technical approach that defines the treatment, and we illustrate our description of the treatment with extensive clinical material. For experienced clinicians, we provide an integrated and, to some degree, innovative synthesis of contemporary psychodynamic approaches to personality pathology and psychodynamic psychotherapy. It is our hope that clinicians will read through and incorporate the approach we describe here and implement it in ways compatible with their individual style, clinical experience, and patient population.

For the reader who wants to pursue a particular topic in greater depth, we provide a selection of recommended readings at the end of each chapter. Where possible, we include both readings that are relatively accessible elaborations on the ideas that we introduce in the preceding chapter and more difficult and sophisticated readings selected because they have significantly contributed to our understanding of a particular topic.

The development of this treatment and this book has been a collaborative effort. We began with a study group, a joint venture of the Personality Disorders Institute of the Sanford Weill Cornell Medical College and the Columbia University Center for Psychoanalytic Training and Research. Participants were (in alphabetical order) Drs. Elizabeth Auchincloss, Eve Caligor, John Clarkin, Diana Diamond, Eric Fertuck, Pamela Foelsch, Otto Kernberg, and Frank Yeomans. Our ideas were further developed in the setting of sharing our approach with candidates at the Columbia University Center for Psychoanalytic Training and Research and with residents at the New York Psychiatric Institute; both groups of students have offered thoughtful questions and critiques that have contributed to the development of the ideas presented in this book.

In addition, we gratefully acknowledge the help of colleagues who have generously offered their time and expertise. Drs. Lucy LaFarge and Steven Roose helped us shape sections of the manuscript along the way, and Drs. Daniel Richter and Bret Rutherford offered thoughtful comments on an earlier draft of this book. Ms. Gina Atkinson has provided editorial assistance.

The reader will find that the chapters in this book are not organized in chronological order, for example beginning with assessment and the opening phase and moving through termination. Instead, we have organized the book and chosen the sequence of chapters to help the reader develop the best possible understanding of the treatment—both of the specific psychotherapeutic technique of DPHP and of the rationale for that technique. Our primary emphasis is not on answering specific questions about "What do I when…" Rather, our aim is to enable the reader to answer for himself the question "How do I systematically go about deciding what to do now?"

The book is divided into three sections. After an introductory chapter, the first section of the book covers our theoretical model of personality and of personality pathology. We begin with a thorough introduction to theory, because a solid understanding of our model of personality pathology and mental functioning is an invaluable, if not essential, foundation for learning how to do the treatment we describe in this volume.

The second section of the book provides an in-depth explication of the treatment. We begin this section with an overview, introducing the basic elements of DPHP and our model for how the treatment works. We next describe the strategies of DPHP, which organize the treatment as a whole, and the treatment setting, which serves as both the stage for and the container of the psychotherapeutic technique that we describe in the chapters that follow. In the final two chapters of this section, we cover the specific technical features of the treatment—the techniques the therapist uses moment to moment in session, and the tactics that guide the therapist in deciding when and how to intervene.

In the third and final section of the book we cover assessment and special situations. Even though treatment begins with assessment, we have opted to place the assessment chapter late in the book, because rational decision making with regard to patient assessment and treatment planning are predicated on a clear understanding of both personality pathology and psychotherapeutic treatment. After covering patient assessment, we circle back to discuss special issues specific to the different phases of treatment. We end with a chapter on combining DPHP with medication management and other forms of treatment.

Before turning to the text, we want to comment on the nature of the clinical material that we present in this book. When writing about the clinical situation, the writer is always torn between the wish to provide actual and true-to-life clinical material and the need to protect patient confidentiality. We have found that, even when patients' identities are disguised, it is impossible to accurately present clinical material while respecting patient confidentiality; at the very least, the patients whose therapy sessions are cited recognize the clinical material. As a result, we have chosen not to present actual patients or actual clinical material in this book. Instead, each clinical vignette that we present is a composite of several patients we have treated and/or whose treatments we have supervised over the years.

Finally, the reader will notice that we use "he" when we might as accurately use "she" or "she or he." While we are not entirely satisfied with this choice, we consistently use male pronouns in order to write as clearly as possible, with the aim of making relatively difficult material easier to read.

ABOUT THE AUTHORS

Eve Caligor, M.D., is Clinical Professor of Psychiatry at the Columbia University College of Physicians and Surgeons in New York City. She is a Training and Supervising Analyst and Director of the Psychodynamic Psychotherapy Division at the Columbia University Center for Psychoanalytic Training and Research in New York City.

Otto F. Kernberg, M.D., is Director of the Personality Disorders Institute at the New York Presbyterian Hospital, Westchester Division, and Professor of Psychiatry at the Joan and Sanford I. Weill Medical College and Graduate School of Medical Sciences of Cornell University, New York City. He is a Training and Supervising Analyst at the Columbia University Center for Psychoanalytic Training and Research and is a past president of the International Psychoanalytic Association.

John F. Clarkin, Ph.D., is Co-Director of the Personality Disorder Institute at New York Presbyterian Hospital, Westchester Division, and Clinical Professor of Psychology in Psychiatry at the Joan and Sanford I. Weill Medical College and Graduate School of Medical Sciences of Cornell University in New York City. He is past president of the International Society for Psychotherapy Research.

CHAPTER 1

INTRODUCTION AND OVERVIEW

This volume describes a psychotherapeutic technique for treating personality pathology. Our aim is to present an approach to psychotherapy that will be of use to seasoned clinicians and can also be used for clinical training. While this book is primarily a textbook of psychotherapeutic technique, dedicated to the psychodynamic clinician, our goal is to present an approach to psychotherapy that is sufficiently systematic, clear, and specific to be useful as a treatment manual (Caligor 2005) in the research setting as well.

In this handbook we present a contemporary psychodynamic approach to understanding and treating the inflexible and maladaptive personality traits that characterize higher level personality pathology. We are describing a relatively long term (1–4 years) twice-weekly psychodynamic treatment. A treatment of this kind cannot be reduced to a series of steps to be followed in a standardized way by any therapist treating any patient. Rather, we define and explicate a series of clinical principles that can be applied in different clinical situations; the treatment we are describing embraces the individual differences as well as the similarities that characterize our patients and the therapists who treat them.

There are a variety of ways to understand personality pathology. The psychodynamic, neurobiological, interpersonal, and cognitive approaches are the most prominent (Lenzenweger and Clarkin 2005). The treatment approach described in this manual is based on a psychodynamic approach to personality, as developed by Kernberg (1975, 1976, 1980, 1984, 1992, 2004a, 2004b), and is heavily influenced by psychodynamic object relations theory. Using this model, Clarkin, Yeomans, and Kernberg have written a manual for the psychodynamic treatment of patients with borderline personality disorder (Clarkin et al. 2006). This book is intended to be a companion to that volume.

THE PATIENTS

Patients with different forms of psychopathology will benefit from different treatment approaches (Beutler et al. 2000). As a result, psychotherapeutic treatments must be tailored to the psychopathology and the psychological assets of the patients being treated. The treatment described in this manual is designed to treat *higher level* personality pathology. Patients who present with this kind of psychopathology constitute a relatively healthy subset of patients within the larger group of patients with personality pathology.

In contrast to the more severe personality disorders emphasized in DSM-IV-TR (American Psychiatric Association 2000), individuals with higher level personality pathology are generally able to adapt to the demands of reality. These individuals benefit from a relatively stable sense of self, a capacity to establish and maintain at least some relationships, and an ability to pursue goals and to work more or less consistently over time. However, people with higher level personality pathology are nonetheless seriously compromised in central areas of functioning. Specifically, these individuals may be unable to establish intimate relations and/or they may find their friendships unsatisfactory. They may be unable to work at a level commensurate with their training and abilities, or they may be compelled to devote themselves entirely to work, to the neglect of relationships and other interests. People with higher level personality pathology may have difficulty asking for help, when they need it, from friends or colleagues, and/or they may find it difficult to make use of help when it is offered. These individuals are unable to function to their full capacity and often suffer from symptoms of anxiety and depression as well as general unhappiness and decreased life satisfaction.

OVERVIEW OF DYNAMIC PSYCHOTHERAPY FOR HIGHER LEVEL PERSONALITY PATHOLOGY (DPHP)

DPHP is a clinical application of contemporary psychodynamic object relations theory designed specifically to treat the rigidity that characterizes higher level personality pathology. Within a psychodynamic frame of reference, personality rigidity and maladaptive personality traits are understood as manifestations of the patient's defensive operations as they interact with temperamental factors. Defenses enable the patient to avoid painful and threatening aspects of his internal life by splitting them off from conscious self-experience. Because defenses serve important functions, patients do not easily gain insight into these defensive operations and the conflicts underlying them.

DPHP is designed to help patients become aware of their defensive operations and psychological conflicts. The overall approach is to establish a special relationship between the therapist and the patient that facilitates the emergence of the patient's conflicts into consciousness, where they are expressed in the patient's relationships, including the relationship with the therapist. Bringing unconscious conflicts into the patient's awareness makes it possible for therapist and patient to work together to help the patient 1) understand the functions served by rigid defensive operations and 2) tolerate emotional awareness of unacceptable aspects of his internal life that have been defensively split off.

To the degree that the patient is able to fully experience conflictual images of himself and others and to assimilate these images into his conscious experience, his need to rigidly maintain defensive operations will be diminished. This process will introduce greater flexibility into the patient's defensive operations, diminish personality rigidity, and deepen and broaden his emotional experience. In DPHP, we do not aim to address all of the patient's conflicts and areas of maladaptive functioning; rather, DPHP focuses on areas of conflict and rigidity associated with the patient's presenting complaints and the treatment goals mutually agreed upon by patient and therapist.

The pace of this work is difficult to predict, and there will be much variability, depending on the degree of rigidity of the patient's defenses, the skill of the therapist, and the readiness and ability of the patient for self-observation. As a result, this handbook cannot tell the reader that a particular intervention will take place in session 4 or session 40. Rather, we offer a set of techniques, based on fundamental clinical principles, and an expected progression and unfolding of the treatment. To make it possible for the reader to learn a treatment of this type, which is somewhat flexible and variable in its course and of relatively long duration, we provide clear descriptions of the goals, strategies, tactics, and techniques of the treatment. A therapist who understands the goals and strategies of the treatment, as well as the model of mental functioning and therapeutic change on which the treatment is built, is in the best possible position to deliver this treatment effectively.

PERSONALITY RIGIDITY, UNCONSCIOUS[1] CONFLICTS, AND INTERNAL OBJECT RELATIONS IN DPHP

Within a psychodynamic frame of reference, psychological conflicts are seen as organized around powerful, highly motivated wishes, needs, or fears, referred to as *conflictual motivations*. Motivations that commonly become involved in conflict include those tied to sexual desire, anger, sadism, competition, power, autonomy, and self-regard, as well as wishes to be loved, admired, or taken care of. In the psychodynamic model, conflictual motivations are kept out of conscious awareness because their expression would be painful or threatening, leading to unpleasant feelings such as anxiety, guilt, fear, depression, or shame. For example, the individual may believe "When I am mean, it makes me a bad person," or "If I turn to someone for love and support, I will be humiliated." Defensive operations that function to keep these potentially threatening motivations out of conscious awareness introduce rigidity into personality functioning.

Conflictual motivations can be conceptualized in terms of wished-for, needed, or feared images of relationships, or *internalized relationship patterns* (Kernberg 1992). In the example, "being mean" might be experienced in terms of a hostile self attacking and damaging someone less strong, while the wish to be taken care of might be represented as a happy, dependent self being nurtured by a caring mother. Personality rigidity resulting from psychological conflict thus can be understood in terms of the need to fend off awareness of painful and threatening internalized relationship patterns and associated affect states.

In psychodynamic object relations theory, internalized relationship patterns are seen as essential organizers of psychological functioning. These relationship patterns are referred to as *internal object relations* and are conceptualized in terms of an image of the self interacting with another person (referred to as an *object*[2]), linked to a particular affect state. It is of interest that other disciplines have developed very similar constructs; attachment theory emphasizes the important role played by *internal working models* as organizers of mental activity (Bretherton 1995; Fonagy 2001); cognitive-

---

[1] The term *unconscious* was used by Sigmund Freud to refer to aspects of psychological experience that are entirely inaccessible to consciousness. This use of the term emphasizes the role of repression and related defenses in psychological life. However, in this volume, we use the term in a more general sense, to refer to all aspects of psychological experience that are currently, defensively, split off from awareness. Thus when we use the term *unconscious* we include not only aspects of internal experience that are repressed, but also thoughts, feelings, and perceptions that are selectively inattended to or whose significance is denied or disavowed.

behavioral theory refers to *cognitive schemas* (Beck et al. 1979; Clark et al. 1999); and cognitive neuroscience views these structures as "associational neural networks" (Gabbard 2001; Westen and Gabbard 2002).

Kernberg (1976) suggests that internal object relations are derived from emotionally invested interactions with significant others that were internalized during development and organized to form enduring memory structures. In this context, the term *structure* refers to a stable, repetitively activated, and enduring pattern of psychological functions that organizes the individual's behavior, perceptions, and subjective experience. Although they are shaped by past relationships, internal object relations do not necessarily have a one-to-one correspondence with actual past interactions with significant others. Instead, internal representations of self and other are seen as reflecting a combination of actual (interpersonal) and fantasied aspects of past relationships, as well as defenses in relation to both aspects. Although internal object relations tend to be relatively stable over time, they are potentially modifiable.

STRATEGIES, TACTICS, AND TECHNIQUES OF DPHP

The *strategies* of a treatment are the overarching principles that organize the treatment *as a whole*, with the aim of meeting the treatment goals. In DPHP, the overarching strategy used to attain the goal of reducing personality rigidity is to bring the internalized relationship patterns underlying the patient's presenting complaints into the treatment so that they can be identified, explored, and worked through. In DPHP, conflictual relationship patterns are worked through in the context of the patient's important current relationships, including the relationship with the therapist. This entire procedure relies both on insight and on the containing functions of the relationship with the therapist. The treatment setting and the psychotherapeutic relationship are both designed specifically to promote emergence of unconscious conflicts and relationship patterns into consciousness.

Tactics are the principles the therapist uses to guide decision making *in each session* with regard to when, where, and how to intervene. In DPHP, the therapist identifies, in each session, the affectively dominant issue expressed in the patient's verbal and nonverbal communication, supplemented by the therapist's emotional experience of his interactions with the patient. Having

---

[2]In psychoanalytic terminology, the word *object* is used, for historical reasons and rather unfortunately, to refer to a person with whom the subject has a relationship. Similarly, the term *internal object* is used to refer to the representation or presence of another within the mind of the subject.

identified the affectively dominant issue, or "priority theme," the therapist makes a link to the dominant unconscious conflict that this theme represents and describes representations of self and other associated with this conflict. Once a conflict is defined, it is systematically explored, moving from conscious aspects of experience to aspects that are less accessible to consciousness, and from defenses to underlying, conflictual relationship patterns. As a conflict comes into focus, the therapist will interpret this conflict in its relation to the patient's presenting complaints and treatment goals.

In any given session in DPHP, the affectively dominant issue may reside in the relationship with the therapist or in a relationship with someone other than the therapist. As treatment progresses, there is often an increasing focus on the relationship with the therapist, and this can be linked to other important relationships, past and present. This triangle (Malan 2004), comprising transference, present relationships, and important relationships from the developmental past, comes to serve as a window into the patient's current internal object relations and unconscious conflicts.

Techniques are the tools a therapist employs in interacting with a patient—the specific methods the therapist uses, *moment to moment* in each session, when listening to the patient and when making an intervention. Techniques employed by the DPHP therapist are containment, making use of countertransference, analysis of resistance, interpretation of psychological conflicts, and a special form of psychotherapeutic "listening." DPHP does not make use of supportive techniques, such as providing encouragement or advice. In DPHP, the use of supportive techniques represents a deviation from technical neutrality.

WHICH TREATMENTS FOR WHICH PATIENTS?

Patients with higher level personality pathology carry a favorable prognosis and are likely to benefit from a variety of psychodynamic treatment approaches, ranging from supportive or short-term focal treatments at one end of the spectrum through psychoanalysis at the other end of the spectrum. Supportive and focal psychodynamically based treatments focus on relatively rapid symptom relief; alteration in the underlying personality is generally not a goal. In contrast, the goal of psychoanalysis is to modify the patient's personality in a relatively comprehensive fashion by providing opportunity to work through all major areas of unconscious conflict in an intensive treatment over the course of many years.

Like psychoanalysis, the treatment described in this manual is designed to modify personality rigidity. However, this treatment is different from psychoanalysis insofar as it is designed to focus on specific areas of conflict and does not rely as heavily on transference interpretation as does psycho-analysis. These modifications of standard psychoanalytic goals and technique are compatible with a treatment of shorter duration (generally 1–4 years) and less intensity (twice-weekly sessions) than psychoanalysis.

Patients with higher level personality pathology who have a concurrent affective or anxiety disorder can benefit from cognitive-behavioral and interpersonal therapies (CBT, IPT) and also short-term psychodynamic psychotherapy (STDP) (Lambert and Ogles 2004), as well as from medication. These treatments have been specifically designed to treat anxiety disorders and depression. STDPs are time-limited treatments based on psychodynamic principles that are organized around a specific symptom, conflict, or relationship pattern. Both CBT and IPT are non-psychodynamic treatments that focus on the individual's patterns of response to environmental stimuli of various kinds. Cognitive-behavioral treatments focus on and attempt to modify repetitive behaviors and patterns of cognition that are maladaptive. Interpersonal psychotherapy focuses on and attempts to modify maladaptive interpersonal patterns and to improve the patient's current interpersonal relations.

The question of what forms of psychotherapy are most appropriate for which patients is an important and controversial one. In our experience, when patients with personality pathology are seen in consultation, decision making is often clouded by confusion between treatment plans that aim to ameliorate symptoms and those that aim to ameliorate maladaptive personality traits. Because many if not most patients with higher level personality pathology presenting for treatment come initially for symptom relief, clear thinking about treatment goals is needed. It is important to formulate a treatment plan that is compatible with the patient's treatment goals, and the therapist must ensure that the patient fully understands and endorses the treatment plan before initiating treatment. In formulating a plan, it is necessary to distinguish between treatments that aim to ameliorate symptoms and DPHP, which aims to ameliorate manifestations of personality rigidity.

We do not believe that DPHP is the most efficient or the best treatment for many of the disorders—such as depressive disorders, anxiety disorders, substance abuse, eating disorders, or sexual dysfunction—that bring patients to treatment. At the same time, it is clear that standard treatments for these disorders are not designed to treat the underlying personality structure in which the disorder is embedded. As a result, for patients with higher level personality pathology who present with symptoms for which there are established treatments with documented efficacy, optimizing treatment will entail explicit discussion of treatment goals and a clear understanding of what available treatments can offer. Often, combining symptomatic treatment with DPHP, either sequentially or concomitantly, will be the most practical solution and the treatment plan best designed to meet the needs of these patients. We discuss combining DPHP with medication management and other forms of therapy in Chapter 11 of this handbook.

Not all patients with personality pathology who present for help are interested in a relatively long-term and intensive treatment such as DPHP, and some patients with relatively mild personality pathology may not need DPHP. The decision as to whether or not to embark on DPHP is a personal one to be made by each patient in ongoing consultation with his therapist. However, for most patients who are interested in treatment for higher level personality pathology, we recommend DPHP. We believe DPHP offers a broad range of patients the opportunity to modify maladaptive personality functioning in ways that can permanently enhance their quality of life.

SUGGESTED READINGS

Clarkin JO, Yeomans FO, Kernberg OF: Psychotherapy for Borderline Personality. Washington, DC, American Psychiatric Publishing, 2006

Gabbard GO: What can neuroscience teach us about transference? Can J Psychoanal 9:1–18, 2001

Kernberg OF: Psychoanalytic object relations theories, in Contemporary Controversies in Psychoanalytic Theory, Techniques, and Their Applications. New Haven, CT, Yale University Press, 2004, pp 26–47

Leichsenring F, Leibing E: The effectiveness of psychodynamic therapy and cognitive behavior therapy in the treatment of personality disorders: a meta-analysis. Am J Psychiatry 160:1223–1232, 2003

Ogden TH: Internal object relations, in Matrix of the Mind: Object Relations and the Psychoanalytic Dialogue (1986). Northvale, NJ, Jason Aronson, 1993, pp 133–165

Rockland L: Supportive Therapy: A Psychodynamic Approach. New York, Basic Books, 1989

Sandler J, Sandler AM: A theory of internal object relations, in Internal Objects Revisited. Madison, CT, International Universities Press, 1998, pp 121–140

THEORETICAL UNDER-STANDING OF HIGHER LEVEL PERSONALITY PATHOLOGY

2

A PSYCHODYNAMIC APPROACH TO PERSONALITY PATHOLOGY

In this chapter we introduce a psychodynamic approach to personality and personality pathology. We describe the psychopathology that dynamic psychotherapy for higher level personality pathology (DPHP) is designed to treat, and we define the population of patients most likely to benefit from this treatment. We focus in particular on the rigidity that characterizes higher level personality pathology, and we describe the clinical presentation of personality rigidity in this population of patients. We also explore the spectrum of defensive operations associated with personality rigidity. We complete the chapter with an introduction to unconscious conflict and to the relationship between unconscious conflict and internal object relations in personality pathology.

PERSONALITY AND PERSONALITY PATHOLOGY

DEFINING PERSONALITY AND PERSONALITY PATHOLOGY

Personality refers to the dynamic organization of enduring patterns of behavior, cognition, emotion, motivation, and ways of relating to others that are characteristic of an individual. An individual's personality is an integral part of his experience of himself and of the world—so much so that he may have difficulty imagining being different. The patterns of behavior, cognition, emotion, and interpersonal relatedness that are organized to comprise an individual's personality are referred to as personality *traits*. Psychodynamic clinicians sometimes use the terms *character* and *character traits* to refer to those aspects of personality that are predominantly psychologically and developmentally determined, in contrast to those that reflect predominantly temperamental factors.

A description of personality will include 1) the nature and the level of organization of personality traits, 2) the degree of flexibility or rigidity with which personality traits are activated across situations, and 3) the extent to which personality traits are adaptive or to which they interfere with functioning and cause distress. A description of personality will also include 4) the nature of the individual's ethical values and ideals, as well as 5) his customary way of adapting (or failing to adapt) to psychosocial stressors. These directly observable components of personality functioning comprise the *descriptive* features of an individual's personality and personality pathology.

In the normal personality, personality traits are not extreme and they are flexibly and adaptively activated in different settings. In this context, we may speak of an individual's having a particular personality "style," for example obsessive-compulsive or histrionic, in the absence of psychopathology. As personality traits become more extreme and more inflexibly activated across situations, we move from normal personality functioning toward increasing degrees of personality pathology until, at the most severe end of the spectrum, personality traits become grossly maladaptive and disruptive of functioning. Regardless of whether personality pathology is relatively mild or more severe, it is by definition associated with some degree of emotional distress and/or impairment in social or occupational functioning. Personality pathology is relatively stable over time, with onset by early adulthood.

The goal of DPHP is to address aspects of personality that are predominantly psychological in origin, reflecting the inflexible and maladaptive activation of the patient's defensive operations. However, it is important to note that not all rigidities of personality are psychologically determined. Rather, many aspects of personality, for example shyness or stimulus seeking, reflect genetically based temperamental factors. In addition, some personality traits that may seem to reflect a rigidity of character, such as a depressive outlook or a tendency toward anxious ruminations, may in fact be the expression of an undiagnosed affective illness or anxiety disorder.

A PSYCHODYNAMIC DESCRIPTION OF PERSONALITY AND PERSONALITY PATHOLOGY

From a psychodynamic perspective, a comprehensive description of personality pathology will include 1) the *descriptive* features of the disorder, 2) a formulation about the *structural* organization underlying descriptive features, and 3) a theory about the patient's *psychodynamics*, which give meaning to the descriptive and structural features of the patient's personality. Assessment of descriptive features provides information about presenting complaints and problems, maladaptive personality traits, and relationships with significant others, and it can be used to formulate a descriptive diagnosis (i.e. the type of diagnosis provided by DSM-IV-TR [American Psychiatric Association 2000]). A structural formulation (described below and also in Chapter 9, "Patient Assessment and Differential Treatment Planning") provides information about the severity of personality pathology through the lens of the individual's experience of himself and his significant others, object relations, defensive operations, and reality testing (Kernberg 1984). Together, descriptive and structural assessments offer the clinician a clear appreciation of the patient's objective and subjective difficulties and provide the information needed to make a diagnosis and to guide treatment planning.

Although descriptive and structural assessments are sufficient to make a diagnosis, a comprehensive psychodynamic description of psychopathology will also include an understanding of the unconscious motivations and psychological conflicts underlying the disorder. This is because psychodynamic models of the mind and treatment embrace the idea that much of what people do and feel is unconsciously motivated. It is by uncovering the unconscious conflicts underlying the patient's manifest feelings and behaviors that the psychodynamic therapist gives meaning to the seemingly irrational difficulties that bring the patient to treatment. And it is through the exploration and working through of underlying meanings and motivations that the psychodynamic therapist will help the patient develop greater flexibility and adaptation.

HIGHER LEVEL PERSONALITY PATHOLOGY

The treatment described in this manual is designed to treat personality rigidity, manifested as inflexible and maladaptive personality traits and associated symptoms, in patients who present with what we refer to as higher level personality pathology. In the section to follow we define this population of patients from three different perspectives. We begin with diagnostic considerations. Next, we elaborate the descriptive features of higher level personality pathology, focusing on the role of maladaptive personality traits. Finally, we discuss how this group of patients can be defined using Kernberg's (1984) psychodynamic, structural approach to classification of personality pathology.

DIAGNOSTIC FEATURES OF HIGHER LEVEL PERSONALITY PATHOLOGY

The patients that DPHP is designed to treat are a relatively healthy sub-population among individuals with personality pathology. Although some meet criteria for a DSM-IV-TR personality disorder, many do not. Instead, the majority of patients with higher level personality pathology present with clinically significant but diagnostically "subthreshold" DSM-IV-TR personality pathology or, alternatively, pathology that is poorly covered in DSM-IV-TR Axis II.

Axis II of DSM-IV-TR provides categorical personality disorder diagnoses. For each personality disorder, personality traits that tend to cluster together in familiar constellations are listed as diagnostic criteria, and the diagnosis of a particular personality disorder is made when the individual meets a specified number of criteria (for example, five of nine for borderline personality disorder). The cutoff for diagnosing any given personality disorder is to some degree arbitrary (i.e., if an individual meets x criteria he has a personality disorder, and if he meets $x-1$ criteria he does not), and the DSM-IV task force selected relatively high diagnostic thresholds (Widiger 1993). The outcome is that many milder forms of personality disorder and personality pathology are poorly covered in DSM-IV-TR Axis II. The poor coverage of various forms of personality pathology provided by the current DSM Axis II classification has received attention elsewhere (Westen and Arkowitz-Westen 1998; Widiger and Mullins-Sweatt 2005).

There is evidence that higher level personality pathology is both common and clinically significant. Westen and Arkowitz-Westen (1998) surveyed a sample of 238 practicing psychiatrists and psychologists, who reported that 60% of patients presenting with clinically significant personality pathology could not be diagnosed by using the DSM-IV-TR classification. There is evidence that subthreshold levels of the DSM personality disorders affect mental health and social adaptation (Skodol et al. 2005; Widiger 1993), and research that views personality pathology as on a continuum with normal personality traits suggests that even somewhat maladaptive personality functioning can adversely influence adaptation and quality of life (Costa and Widiger 1994; Kendler et al. 2004).

Some patients who present with higher level personality pathology meet criteria for one of the DSM-IV-TR personality disorders (Table 2–1). Spe-

---

TABLE 2–1. DSM-IV-TR personality disorders diagnosed in patients with higher level personality pathology

---

Avoidant personality disorder
Dependent personality disorder
Depressive personality disorder (research criteria)
Histrionic personality disorder
Obsessive-compulsive personality disorder

---

cifically, the DSM-IV-TR obsessive-compulsive personality disorder, the depressive personality disorder described in Appendix B of DSM-IV-TR, and a relatively high-functioning subset of patients with DSM-IV-TR histrionic, avoidant, and dependent personality disorders constitute a group of higher level personality disorders within the DSM-IV-TR Axis II classification system. Other patients with higher level personality pathology present with a variety of personality traits listed in DSM-IV-TR Axis II but have an insufficient number of such traits to meet diagnostic criteria for a personality disorder. These patients can be diagnosed as having "subthreshold" personality disorders under the current DSM system or as having personality disorder "traits" if only a few of the listed criteria are present (Oldham and Skodol 2000). Finally, many patients with higher level personality pathology present with maladaptive personality traits that are poorly described in the current DSM-IV-TR diagnostic system yet are commonly encountered in clinical practice. We include here problems with intimacy and commitment, shyness, low self-esteem, devaluation of others, and work inhibitions.

The *Psychoanalytic Diagnostic Manual* (PDM Task Force 2006) provides a contemporary psychoanalytic approach to personality pathology and personality disorders. This manual presents a dimensional perspective on personality pathology currently embraced by many psychoanalytic clinicians, and it also provides a psychodynamically oriented description of the most commonly identified personality disorders. Within this psychoanalytic diagnostic framework, many patients with higher level personality pathology fall into the group of "neurotic personality disorders." The neurotic personality disorders constitute a class of relatively mild personality disorders, on a continuum with the normal personality but characterized by personality styles that are excessively rigid. The most commonly described neurotic personality disorders are the obsessive and/or compulsive personality disorder, the hysterical personality disorder (which is a higher functioning and less extreme version of histrionic personality disorder), and the depressive or depressive-masochistic personality disorder (PDM Task Force 2006).

DESCRIPTIVE FEATURES OF
HIGHER LEVEL PERSONALITY PATHOLOGY

The key observable phenomenon associated with higher level personality pathology is inflexibility or rigidity. Personality rigidity is manifested as a cluster of personality traits or as a particular personality "style" that is inflexibly activated across a variety of situations. Personality rigidity can also be the cause of psychological symptoms. When we speak of *rigidity* in the context of personality pathology, it implies that personality traits are to some degree maladaptive or a cause of distress to the individual with personality pathology and/or the people around him.

When personality traits are rigid, they are automatically and repeatedly activated, regardless of whether they are adaptive or appropriate in a given setting, and efforts to consciously suppress or alter them typically generate anxiety. Personality traits are consistent and stable across situations and through time, and they are resistant to change as a result of experience, learning, new circumstances, or choice. At the least severe end of the spectrum, such personality traits may be ego syntonic; though visible to others, they are typically invisible to the people who exhibit them. In more severe cases of personality rigidity, traits are overtly pathological, and often the individual will sense that certain traits interfere with meeting environmental demands and internal needs. However, even when an individual is aware of and troubled by maladaptive personality traits, he may find that he is unable to change them. Instead, he may watch himself making the same mistakes over and over again, even despite good advice and his own best efforts.

In addition to maladaptive personality traits, higher level personality pathology can be associated with a wide variety of symptoms; these may include physical symptoms, disturbances of mood, disturbances of thought, and abnormal activation or inhibition of behavior. Common examples of physical symptoms that can result from psychological causes include psychogenic fatigue, conversion symptoms, and erectile dysfunction. Emotional symptoms include anxiety and low-grade depression. Common cognitive symptoms that may accompany personality rigidity are hypochondriacal concerns and compulsive and intrusive feelings of regret. Behavioral disturbances include sexual inhibitions and avoidance of situations that might generate anxiety.

CLINICAL ILLUSTRATION OF PERSONALITY RIGIDITY

A young man enjoyed being congenial, and he aimed to please in his interactions with others. He had not been entirely aware of these personality traits, and certainly did not experience them as a problem, until he became a lawyer and was told in his review at work that he needed to be more confrontational in the courtroom. In response, the young man resolved to alter his behavior. Each day, before entering the courtroom, he told himself that he would behave more confrontationally. However, once in the courtroom and faced with an adversary, this young man would invariably feel anxious. The next thing he knew, he would find himself behaving in his usual affable and conciliatory manner.

STRUCTURAL FEATURES OF HIGHER LEVEL PERSONALITY PATHOLOGY

The model of psychopathology and treatment described in this manual is derived from the theory of personality disorders developed by Kernberg (1975, 1976, 1980, 1984, 1992, 2004a, 2004b), based in psychodynamic object relations theory. Kernberg's approach to personality focuses on psychological "structures" thought to underlie the descriptive features of normal personality functioning and personality pathology. In a psychodynamic frame of reference, psychological structures are conceptualized as stable and enduring patterns of psychological functioning that are repetitively activated in particular circumstances. Psychological structures organize an individual's behavior, perceptions, and subjective experience.

In Kernberg's model, internal object relations (introduced in Chapter 1 in the section "Overview of DPHP"), each comprising a representation of the self interacting with the representation of another person and associated with a particular affect state, are the most basic psychological structures. Kernberg suggests that groups of internal object relations that serve related functions are organized to form higher order psychological structures. Kernberg focuses in particular on *identity*, the higher order psychological structure responsible for the individual's sense of self and also for his sense of significant others (Kernberg 2006). Kernberg contrasts normal identity with pathological identity formation, which, following Erikson (1956), he refers to as the syndrome of *identity diffusion* (Akhtar 1992).

In normal identity, internal object relations are integrated and organized to comprise a stable and coherent sense of self in which different aspects of self experience are fluidly activated across different situations and emotional states. In the setting of normal identity, the individual's experience of significant others is also relatively well integrated and stable, and the individual has the capacity to pull together different aspects of another person to comprise a coherent and "whole" image of the other. In contrast, in the syndrome of identity diffusion, internal object relations responsible for the individual's sense of self and significant others are poorly integrated and only loosely organized in relation to one another. The outcome with regard to identity formation is a relatively incoherent and unstable series of contradictory self experiences in the absence of an integrated and consistent "core" sense of self. In the setting of identity diffusion, the individual's experience of significant others is also poorly integrated, fragmented, and unstable.

Kernberg divides the universe of personality pathology into two major groups of disorders, or "levels of personality organization," based on the severity of structural pathology. At the less severe level, patients are characterized by maladaptive personality rigidity in the setting of normal identity. At the more severe level, patients present with extreme and highly maladaptive personality rigidity in the setting of clinically significant identity pathology.

Kernberg further distinguishes patients with normal, or consolidated, identity from those with identity pathology on the basis of the nature of their dominant defensive operations and the stability of their reality testing (Table 2–2). In sum, in the healthier group, we see maladaptive personality rigidity in the setting of 1) normal identity, 2) the predominance of higher level, repression-based[1] defensive operations, and 3) intact reality testing. These features define the "neurotic level of personality organization" (NPO) in Kernberg's classification system. In the more severe group, patients present with severely maladaptive personality rigidity in the setting of 1) clinically significant identity pathology, 2) the predominance of lower level, splitting-based, defensive operations, and 3) variable reality testing in which ordinary reality testing is grossly intact but the more subtle capacity to accurately perceive the inner states of others is impaired. These features define the "borderline level of personality organization" (BPO).[2]

Although Table 2–2 presents Kernberg's classification of neurotic and borderline levels of personality organization in a categorical format, in practice, this diagnostic system provides a dimensional assessment of personality pathology. At the healthiest end of the spectrum are individuals with normal identity, predominantly higher level defenses, and stable reality testing; at the most severe end of the spectrum are those with severe identity pathology, predominantly lower level defenses, and shaky reality

---

[1] We discuss classification of defensive operations and the role of repression and splitting-based defenses in personality pathology later in this chapter.

[2] We want to make clear the distinction between the DSM-IV-TR borderline personality disorder (BPD) and the borderline level of personality organization (BPO). BPD is a specific personality disorder, diagnosed on the basis of a constellation of descriptive features. BPO is a much broader category based on structural features—in particular, pathology of identity formation. The BPO diagnosis subsumes the DSM-IV-TR BPD, as well as all of the severe personality disorders. We refer the reader to Figure 2–1 for further clarification of the relationship between the DSM-IV-TR Axis II diagnostic categories and level of personality organization.

TABLE 2–2. Structural diagnosis: three levels of personality organization

	Level of personality organization		
	Normal	**Neurotic**	**Borderline**
Identity	Consolidated	Consolidated	Poorly consolidated
Defenses	Mature defenses predominate	Repression-based defenses predominate	Splitting-based defenses predominate
Rigidity	Flexible adaptation	Rigidity	Severe rigidity
Reality testing	Intact and stable	Intact and stable	Essentially intact but deteriorates in the setting of affective intensity Capacity to accurately read the inner states of others is compromised

testing. In between, we find a range of psychopathology. This is to say that Kernberg's classification is most accurately conceptualized as describing a continuous spectrum of personality pathology, based on pathology of identity formation, defensive operations, and reality testing. As a result, the demarcation between the neurotic and borderline levels of personality organization is not categorical, and there are patients with very mild identity pathology who present with mixed features.

Kernberg's classification system, based on severity of pathology of object relations, can be combined with DSM-IV-TR Axis II to locate personality pathology in two-dimensional space, as illustrated in Figure 2–1. Higher level personality pathology as we have defined it corresponds with Kernberg's neurotic level of personality organization, as well as with personality pathology that falls at the transition between the NPO and BPO levels (i.e., patients with mild identity pathology who rely on a combination of higher level and lower level defenses). In contrast, the majority of patients with DSM-IV-TR personality disorders fall into Kernberg's borderline level of personality organization.

IDENTITY IN THE CLINICAL SETTING

Normal identity is associated with an experience of self and significant others that is continuous over time and across situations, and with a capacity to appreciate the attributes and the inner experience of others in a way that

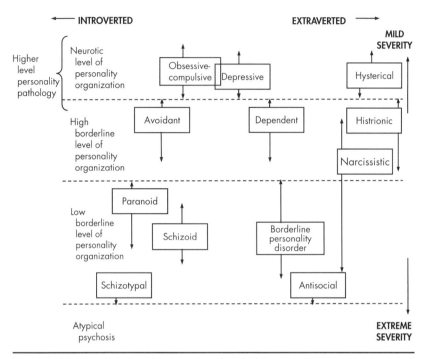

FIGURE 2–1. Relationship between level of personality organization and DSM-IV-TR Axis II diagnoses.

Severity ranges from mildest, at the top of the diagram, to extremely severe, at the bottom. Vertical arrows indicate ranges of severity for each DSM-IV-TR personality disorder.

conveys complexity, subtlety, and depth. Normal identity is also associated with the capacity to invest, over time, in professional, intellectual, and recreational interests and to "know one's mind" with regard to one's own values, opinions, tastes, and beliefs. The treatment described in this manual is intended for patients who present with personality pathology in the setting of relatively well consolidated identity. Our psychotherapeutic technique is predicated on the patient's having essential psychological capacities that are associated with identity consolidation and that may be impaired in patients with clinically significant identity pathology. We include here the capacity to commit to and invest in a long-term treatment, a fairly well developed capacity for self-observation and self-reflection, a capacity to establish and maintain a therapeutic relationship with relative ease, an appreciation of the symbolic nature of thought, and adequate impulse control.

Patients with clinically significant identity pathology present with a markedly different experience of themselves and of the world. Clinically significant identity pathology is associated with a sense of self and an experience of significant others that is fragmented and unstable across time and across situations. The individual's subjective experience of others tends to be poorly differentiated, lacking in subtlety and depth, and to be more or less polarized ("black and white") and/or superficial. Tastes, opinions, and values are inconsistent, typically adopted from others in the environment, and they may shift easily and dramatically with changes in milieu. The individual with identity pathology often lacks a capacity to accurately "read" others and may be unable to respond tactfully and appropriately to subtle social cues. Poorly consolidated identity is typically associated with a paucity of meaningful investments in professional, intellectual, and recreational pursuits. While most clearly evident in the DSM-IV-TR borderline personality disorder, some degree of identity pathology characterizes all of the severe personality disorders. In the clinical setting, identity pathology is typically associated with a high rate of treatment dropout, an impaired capacity for self-reflection, difficulty in maintaining a therapeutic alliance, a tendency for concrete thinking with the possibility of transient compromise of reality testing, and a tendency for impulsive acting out.

PERSONALITY RIGIDITY

Higher level personality pathology exists on a continuum with the normal personality. In both groups we see identity consolidation in the setting of intact and stable reality testing. However, where in the normal personality we see adaptive and flexible personality functioning, in higher level personality pathology we see maladaptive personality rigidity.

Personality traits are in part made up of constellations of specific defenses that the individual tends to use automatically and repetitively in particular circumstances. The adaptive and flexible functioning seen in the normal personality reflects the flexibility of "healthy" or "mature" defensive operations. Similarly, the rigidity that characterizes higher level personality pathology reflects the relative inflexibility of predominant defensive operations; in addition to the flexible and adaptive defensive operations characteristic of the normal personality, individuals with higher level personality pathology rely on repression-based "neurotic-level" defenses in conjunction with splitting-based "image-distorting" defensive operations. It is the relative stability and inflexibility of neurotic and image-distorting defenses as they are employed in the setting of identity consolidation that is responsible for higher level personality rigidity.

In contrast, in more severe personality pathology (i.e., Kernberg's borderline level of personality organization, comprising the majority of the DSM-IV-

TR Axis II personality disorders; see Figure 2–1), we see personality rigidity in the setting of identity pathology. Personality rigidity in the setting of identity pathology is characterized by extremely maladaptive, contradictory, unstable, and often socially inappropriate behavior patterns and personality traits.

INHIBITORY AND REACTIVE PERSONALITY TRAITS

In higher level personality pathology, maladaptive personality traits may present as inhibitions of normal behaviors ("inhibitory behavior patterns") or as exaggeration of certain behaviors ("reactive" behavior patterns), and many patients present with a combination of the two. In the case of *inhibitory* personality traits, we see the absence of behavior patterns that might be expected or appropriate in a given situation. For example, an individual with conflicts around competitive aggression might adopt a general attitude of passivity, both in his personal and his professional life. This individual is likely to be seen by others as weak and unreliable, someone who will not "step up to the plate" even when called upon to do so and even when he would like to do so. In the case of *reactive* personality traits, we see the presence of behavior patterns that are not necessarily appropriate for a given situation. Returning to our example, instead of being passive, this same person might habitually need to be in control of everything and everyone he is involved with. This individual is likely to spend much of his time worried and anxious, and he may be repeatedly surprised when he discovers that others are alienated by his controlling behavior. However, even when he tries to step back he finds himself unable to do so.

The inhibitory and reactive personality traits seen in personality pathology can be contrasted with the *sublimatory* personality traits typical of the normal personality. In sublimation, conflictual motivations are directed in a manner that is adaptive and constructive, as well as relatively flexible, into nonconflictual areas of functioning. If we return to the example above, an individual with normal personality might address conflicts involving competitive aggression by habitually assuming an attitude that is assertive, effective, and forceful. This individual is likely to be admired by others and to be seen as someone who is successful and can be counted on. Further, in settings in which it might be inappropriate to be assertive, the normal personality would be able to control his wishes to be more assertive, and to modify his behavior accordingly.

CLINICAL PRESENTATION OF PERSONALITY RIGIDITY IN HIGHER LEVEL PERSONALITY PATHOLOGY

Personality rigidity in the setting of higher level personality pathology manifests itself as an inability to adapt smoothly to internal and external sources of anxiety or conflict ("stressors"). In some people, rigidity manifests as a difficulty in "rolling with the punches" or "laughing things off." Rather, when things go wrong or not as planned, these individuals tend to worry excessively and unproductively. They often continue thinking about a problem or disappointment even when there is nothing more to be done, finding it difficult to just "let it go" or "sleep on it." These people often need to feel "in control," and as a result, when faced with a problem, they often tend to blame themselves. Further, they have difficulty letting things come as they will or giving up on something or changing course midstream.

Alternatively, higher level personality rigidity may present as a "breezy" neglect of unpleasant emotions associated with painful or conflictual situations. Painful emotions and the circumstances that stimulate them may be only transiently experienced and then forgotten, or even entirely overlooked. These people may fail to be aware of or take responsibility for their impact on others. Rather than ruminating about a problem, people in this group are likely to forget that it exists or to rationalize that it is unimportant, and to insist in the face of stressful or conflictual situations that everything is fine.

Other common manifestations of the rigidity of higher level personality pathology are inhibitions in relation to sexuality, intimacy, and professional success. These areas of less than optimal functioning typically are a cause of frustration and disappointment for individuals who, despite their best efforts, may find themselves unable to make changes in these areas. Inhibitions may present in the form of distorted self-appraisal in areas of conflict. For example, a patient may think of himself as not particularly successful when he *is* highly successful, or he may view himself as unattractive when in fact he is extremely so. In general, patients with higher level personality rigidity often have difficulty seeing themselves entirely as others see them, typically holding onto an unduly negative or childlike view of themselves, despite years of external feedback to the contrary.

CLINICAL ILLUSTRATIONS OF PERSONALITY RIGIDITY IN HIGHER LEVEL PERSONALITY PATHOLOGY

A professional woman, conflicted about pursuing her own needs over those of others and a perfectionist about her work as a financial advisor, was having difficulty getting pregnant. Much as she vowed to herself and to her therapist that she would keep her appointments with her infertility doctor in the face of her busy work schedule, whenever clients' needs conflicted, she felt anxious until she canceled her doctor's appointment. This highly valued employee always did the best job she possibly could, and she could not imagine doing otherwise. Even so, she frequently doubted her level of performance and was in a chronic state of anxiety that her superiors would see her as a "slacker."

Another patient, an associate in a large law firm, routinely felt anxious and overwhelmed when confronted with difficult situations in her personal life. She tried to deal with her anxiety by asking her husband to reassure her, repeatedly, that everything would turn out fine. In doing this the patient felt irrational and childlike, but when she tried to restrict her requests for reassurance, she felt very uneasy. Despite her professional successes, in her personal life this patient felt of little value—in her own words, "dispensable"—despite the love and open admiration of her husband and children.

A businessman, in therapy for a year and in love for the first time, realized that he became depressed and anxious whenever things became more tender or intimate with his girlfriend. He was able to predict that this would happen but was unable to prevent it. At these times he would go into a panic, worrying that his girlfriend might be losing interest in him or flirting with other men. This fear was exacerbated by his difficulty maintaining an erection during intercourse.

Patients with higher level personality pathology will present with some combination of the kinds of behaviors, thoughts, and feelings that we have described. Most commonly, patients seen in consultation complain of symptoms of anxiety or depression in conjunction with difficulties maintaining long-term, intimate relationships or living up to their full potential at work. Perhaps the most common initial presentation is of someone who is professionally successful and has satisfying friendships but is unable to form a long-term intimate relationship with a partner. These patients want to be married, but they find themselves unable to attain this goal. Not infrequently, patients falling into this group also have sexual symptoms.

Another common presentation is that of a patient who performs well at work but feels something is holding him back or interfering with his fully pursuing his ambitions or living up to his potential. Some patients in this group may be extremely successful yet unable to fully enjoy or "own" their successes. Often, patients presenting with difficulties related to work have problems working easily and effectively with their superiors or have troubled peer relations in the workplace. Patients presenting with work-related problems may or may not also have sexual symptoms or problems in sustaining long-term relationships.

DEFENSIVE OPERATIONS AND PERSONALITY RIGIDITY

Defenses are an individual's automatic psychological responses to internal or external stressors or emotional conflict (Perry and Bond 2005). All defensive operations function to alter subjective experience in order to avoid emotional distress. Although we present here a list of commonly described defense mechanisms, it is generally agreed that the ways in which an individual can defensively organize his internal and external experience are limitless. It is also generally agreed that defenses can be grouped and hierarchically ranked; at one end of the spectrum are the healthiest defenses that are most flexible and adaptive, at the other end of the spectrum are the most pathological defenses that are highly inflexible and maladaptive (Perry and Bond 2005; Vaillant 1992). Defenses at the most adaptive end of the spectrum involve little or no distortion of internal or external reality, and as defenses become more rigid and maladaptive they involve increasing degrees of distortion of reality (Vaillant 1992).

There is a fair amount of agreement among researchers with regard to how defenses can be grouped and hierarchically ranked on the basis of level of adaptation (Perry and Bond 2005). This consensus is represented in the Defensive Functioning Scale in Appendix B of DSM-IV-TR. Kernberg (1976) has presented an approach to the classification of defenses that divides them into three groups: 1) mature defenses, 2) repression-based or "neurotic" defenses, and 3) splitting-based or "primitive" defenses. This classification is in many ways consistent with current consensus within the research community[3] while placing greater emphasis on the psychological mechanisms underlying defensive operations (Table 2–3).

Mature, or healthy, defenses involve minimal distortion of internal and external reality and are associated with the flexible and adaptive functioning of the normal personality. Neurotic-level defenses avoid distress by repressing, or banishing from consciousness, aspects of the subject's psychological experience that are conflictual or a potential source of emotional discomfort. "Primitive," or image-distorting, defenses do not banish mental contents from consciousness per se, but instead compartmentalize, or maintain a distance between, conscious mental contents that are in conflict with each other or whose approximation would generate psychological discomfort (Kernberg 1976).

In higher level personality pathology, neurotic-level and image-distorting defenses automatically and fixedly keep certain aspects of internal and external experience split off from conscious awareness, and this process introduces rigidity into personality functioning.

---

[3] The Defensive Functioning Scale in Appendix B of DSM-IV-TR refers to mature defenses as "high adaptation level" of defenses and to neurotic defenses as "mental inhibitions (compromise formation) level" of defenses. Splitting-based, or image-distorting, defenses as they are defined by Kernberg are divided into "minor image-distorting level" and "major image-distorting level" in DSM-IV-TR.

TABLE 2–3. Classification of defenses

Mature defenses: healthy adaptation and coping

    Suppression

    Anticipation

    Altruism

    Humor

    Sublimation

Neurotic (repression-based) defenses: conflictual aspects of internal experience are banished from consciousness

    Repression

    Reaction formation

    Neurotic projection

    Displacement

    Isolation of affect

    Intellectualization

Image-distorting (splitting-based) defenses: aspects of conscious experience are dissociated to avoid conflict

    Splitting

    Primitive idealization

    Devaluation

    Projective identification

    Omnipotent control

    Primitive denial

Note that image-distorting defenses are often referred to as "primitive" defenses in the psychodynamic literature.

MATURE DEFENSES: ADAPTATION AND COPING

Mature defenses are best described as adaptive and flexible coping mechanisms that enable the individual to deal with anxiety-provoking situations with a minimum of emotional distress (Vaillant 1993). Mature defenses do not bar any aspect of a conflict from consciousness, nor do they maintain a distance between aspects of emotional life that are in conflict. Mature defenses allow all aspects of an anxiety-provoking situation into subjective awareness, with little or no distortion but in a fashion that optimizes coping. Suppression, anticipation, altruism, humor, and sublimation are examples of mature defenses. *Suppression* involves intentionally and adaptively putting aside a particular thought or feeling until a time when constructive action can be taken. *Anticipation* involves planning ahead as a way to deal with potentially stressful situations. *Altruism* involves deriving satisfaction vicariously through helping others. *Humor* involves the capacity to see the comic aspects of a stressful situation, as a way to reduce discomfort and to create useful distance from immediate events. *Sublimation* involves the constructive and creative redirection of conflictual motivations into nonconflictual areas of functioning and is a central feature of normal adaptation.

NEUROTIC DEFENSES: CONFLICTUAL ASPECTS OF INTERNAL EXPERIENCE ARE BANISHED FROM CONSCIOUSNESS

Neurotic defenses all rely to some degree on repression; some aspect of the subject's experience is split off and barred access to consciousness (Kernberg 1976). In classical definitions of repression, the conflictual thought or idea is repressed, although the affect may remain conscious. Thus, a person repressing anger at his spouse will not remember their argument or why he is angry but may feel unexplained irritability on his way home from work. In other forms of repression, the affect may be repressed while the idea remains conscious. Here, a person may express his dissatisfaction to his spouse in a highly rational and emotionally controlled fashion, with no awareness of having powerful feelings tied to the content of his discourse. Alternatively, the affect and the thought may both be repressed, replaced by defensive behavior patterns. Here, a person may automatically and habitually withhold the expression of endearments to his wife, or he may be excessively expressive of his affection—in either case with no awareness of harboring angry or critical thoughts or feelings toward her.

Despite the various forms that repressive defenses can take, all neurotic-level defenses involve repressing or banishing from consciousness some aspect of subjective experience. In *classical repression*, it is the idea that is repressed, whereas in *isolation of affect*, it is the affect that is repressed. *Intellectualization* is similar to isolation—affect is repressed while the individual consciously focuses on abstract ideas. In *reaction formation*, both the affect and the idea vanish and are replaced by their opposites. In *neurotic projection*, it is the connection between the subject and his motives and feelings that is repressed, and in *displacement*, the connection between a motive or feeling and a particular object is repressed. *Rationalization* supports repression by providing seemingly rational explanations for behaviors that have unconscious roots.

In sum, neurotic-level defenses all avoid unpleasant feelings, such as anxiety, depression, shame, guilt, and fear, by repressing or keeping out of awareness aspects of the subject's psychological experience that are conflictual or a potential source of emotional discomfort. As such, neurotic-level defenses alter the subject's internal reality, but they typically do so without grossly distorting the subject's sense of external reality. While neurotic-level defenses are responsible for personality rigidity, influencing cognitive processes and leading to subtle distortions of experience, and may cause discomfort or distress, they typically do not lead to grossly abnormal or disruptive behaviors. In psychotherapy, neurotic-level defenses present as personality traits and character defenses and as unintentional omissions or disruptions in the flow of the patient's communications.

IMAGE-DISTORTING DEFENSES: ASPECTS OF CONSCIOUS EXPERIENCE ARE DISSOCIATED TO AVOID CONFLICT

Where neurotic-level defenses make use of repression, image-distorting defenses make use of dissociation, or "splitting," to avoid psychological conflict and emotional distress.[4] When we use the terms *dissociation* and *splitting* we refer to a psychological process in which two aspects of experience that are in conflict are both allowed to emerge fully into consciousness, but either not at the same time as, or not in conjunction with, the same object relation (Kernberg 1976). For example, a woman may be assertive and effective in her professional life but excessively submissive and passive in her marriage. What we see as a result of image-distorting defenses is that conflicting motivations and aspects of self experience are compartmentalized or "split" apart. Thus, although nothing is repressed when dissociative defenses are employed, conflicting aspects of psychological experience are not simultaneously experienced in relation to the self, and in this process conflict is avoided.

In the psychodynamic literature, the terms *dissociation* and *splitting* are often used more or less interchangeably. *Splitting* is used most frequently when referring to the dissociation of idealized and persecutory, or loving and hateful, aspects of experience, while *dissociation* is more frequently used when referring to the keeping apart of other aspects of self-experience (e.g., sexual and dependent motivations) that are in conflict.

The splitting-based defenses were first systematically described by Melanie Klein (1946, 1952) and include—in addition to splitting proper—idealization, devaluation, projective identification, omnipotent control, and primitive denial. Klein suggested that the predominance of this con-

---

[4]We want to make clear that dissociation as a defensive operation is to be distinguished from dissociative states, which involve the enactment of complex mental experiences in the context of some degree of reduction of consciousness. Dissociative states involve the defensive operation of dissociation, but they also involve an altered state of consciousness; dissociation as a defensive operation does not involve an altered state of consciousness.

stellation of defensive operations is a central feature of what she referred to as the "paranoid schizoid position," a level of psychological development and mental organization that she viewed as quite primitive and characteristic of patients with severe psychopathology. As a result, she referred to the group of splitting-based defenses as *primitive defenses*, and she contrasted them with the classical neurotic defenses that are based on repression.

Many of Klein's ideas remain useful and are consistent with advances in theoretical and empirical study of the severe personality disorders (Kernberg and Caligor 2005; Lenzenweger et al. 2001), and the construct of primitive defenses remains central to Kernberg's (1975) construct of borderline level of personality organization. However, since the time of Klein's original contributions, there has been increasing recognition that even though splitting-based defenses are characteristic of the more severe personality disorders, a variety of splitting-based and dissociative defenses are routinely employed in higher level personality pathology as well (Bion 1962b; Joseph 1987; LaFarge 2000; Rangell 1982; Steiner 1992).

SPLITTING AND DISSOCIATION IN SEVERE PERSONALITY DISORDERS

Kernberg (1984) suggests that splitting (which he also refers to as *primitive dissociation*) is the prototypical defense seen in patients with severe personality disorders, who tend to compartmentalize experiences of self and other that are in conflict. In this group of patients, splitting most commonly pertains to the mutual dissociation of positively colored, idealized sectors of experience and negatively colored, persecutory aspects of experience. What we see as a result are object relations that are experienced as either "all good" or "all bad"—loving, gratifying, and secure on the one hand, or aggressive, frustrating, and frightening on the other.

Projective identification involves splitting off aspects of one's internal experience and projecting them into another person, so that the projected aspects of the self are experienced as part of the other person. At the same time, the individual using projective identification will interact with the other person to elicit responses that are consistent with what has been projected. (This is to say that in projective identification, projections tend to be actualized.) *Idealization* is a form of splitting that involves seeing others as all good in order to avoid anxieties associated with negative feelings. Idealization is often followed by its opposite, *devaluation*. In *omnipotent control*, a grandiose self magically controls a depreciated, emotionally degraded other. *Primitive denial* supports splitting, by maintaining a disregard for aspects of the internal or external world that are either contradictory or potentially threatening. When primitive denial is employed, the individual is cognitively aware of a threatening experience but this awareness fails to evince the corresponding emotional reaction.

In the severe personality disorders, splitting-based defenses are responsible for experiences of self and other that are widely polarized, unrealistic, superficial, and highly affectively charged. Further, splitting-based defenses in the setting of identity pathology are typically unstable and often lead to a rapid and rather chaotically shifting experience of idealized and persecutory experiences of self and other (Kernberg 1984). In this way, primitive defenses cause flagrant distortion of interpersonal reality. In addition, primitive defenses typically have behavioral manifestations and frequently result in disruptive behaviors in the individual with severe personality pathology.

SPLITTING AND DISSOCIATION IN HIGHER LEVEL PERSONALITY PATHOLOGY

Defenses based on splitting and dissociation also play an important role in higher level personality pathology and its treatment. However, in contrast to the situation in the severe personality disorders, we are now seeing the impact of splitting and dissociation on the psychological experience of an individual who has a consolidated identity and a relatively well integrated sense of self. In this setting, what we see most commonly is the dissociation, or splitting off from the dominant sense of self, of motivations and aspects of self experience that are conflictual. As in the severe personality disorders, in higher level pathology, splitting and dissociation are supported by denial; the individual denies the significance of dissociated aspects of conscious experience that are incompatible with his dominant sense of self.

In higher level personality pathology, splitting and dissociation are less extreme and more stable than in more severe personality pathology and typically do not lead to the highly polarized, rapidly shifting, and affectively charged experiences of internal and external reality characteristic of the severe personality disorders. Thus, in higher level personality pathology, splitting and dissociation are not typically associated with "primitive" mental states, but rather with the segregation of aspects of psychological experience that are in conflict and with the more or less subtle dissociation of conflictual motivations from dominant self experience. Specifically, in higher level personality pathology, splitting-based defensive operations are most commonly responsible for personality rigidity and for overly simplified, somewhat one-dimensional versions of experience in which motivations and views of the self that are in conflict are not experienced simultaneously.

CLINICAL ILLUSTRATION OF SPLITTING-BASED DEFENSES IN HIGHER LEVEL PERSONALITY PATHOLOGY

As a commonly encountered example of splitting-based defensive operations at play in higher level personality pathology, we can consider the married man with sexual conflicts. This man might use repression-based defenses to avoid his sexual conflicts, for example, projecting his sexual desire into his wife while experiencing himself as lacking in desire and submitting to her sexual needs. Alternatively, he could use defenses based on dissociation to split off sexual object relations, on the one hand, from tender and dependent object relations, on the other. For example, this man might enjoy sexual relations with his wife only when on vacation in a hotel room far from home and children, while remaining sexually impotent at home. In this case, we would say that this patient has dissociated his sexual relationship with his wife from his dependent and familial relations with her. Alternatively, such a man might reserve all his sexual activity for his mistress, toward whom he feels no tenderness, while maintaining a loving but asexual relationship with his wife. Further, he might deny that his relationship with his mistress is of any consequence, seeing it "simply" as a way to satisfy his sexual appetites and having nothing to do with his relationship with his wife. In this case, we could say that the patient has dissociated tenderness and sexuality by virtue of enacting them in the settings of different relationships. In either case, whether this man has sexual relations only with his wife on vacation or only with his mistress, he will have avoided whatever feelings of anxiety, guilt, shame, or fear are associated in his mind with the experiencing of sexual motivations and tender motivations both at the same time toward the same person.

UNCONSCIOUS CONFLICT

In a psychodynamic frame of reference, maladaptive personality traits and psychological symptoms are understood as reflecting an interaction between inborn temperamental dispositions and unconscious conflicts whose origins lie in the subject's personal history. From birth onward, affectively charged interactions with significant others, colored by temperamental factors, are internalized to form internalized relationship patterns, or internal object relations. Internalized relationship patterns that represent areas of conflict are actively kept out of awareness by the individual's defensive operations and are split off from the person's conscious self experience.[5] Thus, defenses protect the individual from awareness of painful or threatening aspects of his inner life, but at the expense of developing personality rigidity (and sometimes symptoms as well). In the end, it is the individual's difficulty tolerating awareness of and accepting certain aspects of his conscious and unconscious psychological experience that lead to the rigidity that characterizes the higher level personality pathology.

CONFLICT AND STRUCTURE

As described in Chapter 1 ("Introduction and Overview"), unconscious conflicts are organized around powerful wishes, needs, and fears—referred to as *conflictual motivations*, or in classical psychoanalytic terminology as *impulses*—which are kept out of conscious awareness or dissociated from the dominant sense of self because their expression would be painful, threatening, or morally unacceptable to the individual. In addition to a conflictual wish, need, or fear, an unconscious conflict is composed of defensive operations designed to avoid awareness or expression of the conflictual motivation. Painful affects—including guilt, loss, anxiety, fear, depression, and shame—are associated with enactment of conflictual object relations, and these negative affects function to motivate defense.

Conflictual motivations are experienced as wished-for, needed, or feared images of relationships and are mentally represented as highly emotionally charged internalized relationship patterns, or internal object relations (Kernberg 1992), comprising an image of the self interacting with an image of another person. Typically, it is erotic, exhibitionistic, loving, dependent, aggressive, competitive, self-promoting, and sadistic internal object relations that are involved in psychological conflict. Because enactment of these highly affectively charged relationship patterns is associated with painful affects, object relations associated with conflictual motivations are either repressed or dissociated and are not part of the individual's dominant sense of self.

Like conflictual motivations, defenses and anxieties are also experienced and represented as internalized relationship patterns, or internal object relations (Kernberg 1992). What we see clinically is that enactment of defensive relationship patterns functions to keep conflictual object relations out of awareness or dissociated from the dominant sense of self. For example,

---

[5]We wish to clarify that when we speak of internal object relations as split off from dominant *self experience*, we are referring to the splitting off not only of aspects of the individual's sense of self but also of aspects of his experience of the world around him, in order to avoid conflict and negative affect. This is to say that self experience, closely tied to the construct of identity, is determined by one's representations of others as well as by self representations. Thus, when we speak of dominant self experience, we include both the individual's view of himself and also of the world he lives in, including his significant others. For example, in responses to conflicts involving aggression, one may defensively split off awareness of one's own angry feelings ("I am not a hostile person") and/or one may split off awareness of anger in one's objects ("I do not experience hostility from the people I love").

consider the young woman who presents with sexual inhibitions and problems with intimacy. For this woman, sexual excitement is a conflictual motivation that is linked to an internalized relationship pattern of a sexually seductive girl in relation to an excited paternal figure. Because it is morally unacceptable, this erotic object relation is repressed. Further, ongoing repression of this erotic object relation is tied to activation and enactment of a defensive relationship pattern—for example, of a sexually indifferent girl and a nurturing parental figure. This defensive object relation will be experienced consciously and will be part of the patient's dominant sense of self. The patient's experience of herself as a sexually indifferent girl in relation to a nurturing paternal figure is likely to color her romantic experience, as well as her experience of her therapist early in treatment.

In addition to a conflictual motivation and defenses, an unconscious conflict is also composed of object relations signifying the "dangers" associated with enactment of conflictual motivations. Anticipated dangers are linked to negative affects—typically anxiety, guilt, loss, depression, fear, or shame—which function to motivate defense. The constellation of negative affects associated with unconscious conflicts that motivate defense are sometimes referred to as *signal affects* or as the "anxiety" associated with the conflict, and they are sometimes referred to as the *motivation for defense*. While this may sound a bit abstract, in practice, affects and relationship patterns signifying the dangers associated with expression of conflictual motivations can be quite easy to identify in the clinical setting.

To illustrate this point, let's return to the patient described immediately above who has conflicts involving repressed sexual desires. For this patient, we might discover that the affects motivating defense are depression and loss, associated with an internal object relation of a disapproving and rejecting mother and a young girl who feels unloved. Whenever the conflictual motivation begins to break through the defense, that is, whenever this patient perceives the possibility of sexual excitement, she will inexplicably find herself feeling depressed and lonely. This affective experience corresponds with the activation of an internal relationship pattern of a rejecting mother and a lonely child. Not infrequently, only the affect will be conscious to the patient, who remains unaware of the link between her affect state, repressed sexual desires, and a fantasied rejection by a maternal figure. In treatment, feelings of loneliness and depression might be noted by the therapist (if not by the patient) to follow on the heels of meeting a new man. These "signal affects" (Freud 1959 [1926]) will be linked to the possibility of sexual excitement and to the activation of a painful relationship pattern with a rejecting maternal figure.

CLINICAL ILLUSTRATION OF UNCONSCIOUS CONFLICT

In the opening phase of her therapy, a patient established an idealized view of her therapist, much as she maintained an idealized view of her mother and her husband. This internalized relationship pattern, of a well cared-for child and a loving caretaker, was associated with an affective experience of warmth, reassurance, and safety. This conscious experience served a defensive function, protecting the patient from awareness of a different experience of putting herself in the hands of a caretaker. In the course of treatment, an image of a hurt and neglected child and a critical, selfish, and competitive mother began to emerge in the treatment, associated with feelings of anger and fear on the part of the patient. The patient came to be aware of anxiety at the possibility of seeing both the therapist and her current boss in this way, and she also recalled childhood memories of experiences with her parents in which they seemed critical or selfish.

As these anxieties were worked through and the patient became more able to tolerate awareness of negative aspects of the people she relied on, she started to develop an awareness of her own critical, competitive, and selfish feelings, directed toward her mother, her boss, and ultimately her therapist. Initially, as the patient began to be vaguely aware of her own critical, competitive, and selfish feelings, she found herself feeling anxious and guilty, affects that the therapist helped her relate to an image of herself as a bad child who was rightfully going to be criticized and punished. As these anxieties were explored and worked through, the patient became better able to tolerate the formerly unconscious images of herself as competitive, critical, and selfish.

As a result of exploring and working through this patient's conflicts involving her critical, competitive, and selfish feelings, she no longer needed to rigidly idealize caretakers and people in authority, nor did she need to bend over backwards to avoid her own critical and competitive feelings. She became more overtly competitive and more able to see and tolerate the selfish, critical, and competitive aspects of people around her.

OBJECT RELATIONS AND DEFENSE: "LAYERING" AND "ROLE REVERSAL"

In Chapter 3 ("Internal Object Relations, Mental Organization, and Subjective Experience in Personality Pathology"), we will discuss the relationship between internal object relations and defense in greater detail, but we would like to touch on the topic at this point. The clinical example just provided illustrates two different ways in which enactment of internal object relations can serve defensive functions. First, in this vignette, the patient's conscious experience of a well cared-for child and a loving caretaker supports repression of a neglectful caretaking relationship. In classical terminology, we might think of this as a process involving a combination of splitting or idealization and repression. At the same time, within an object relations theory frame of reference, this process could be conceptualized in terms of the layering of internal object relations, such that enactment of a defensive object relation supports repression of underlying internal object relations that are more threatening and, typically, closer to the expression of conflictual motivations.

Second, the patient's initial experience of others as critical, selfish, and competitive protected her against an awareness of critical, selfish, and competitive feelings within herself. This defensive operation, embedded within a single object relation, can be described in terms of the projection of aggressive impulses. We would add that in an object relations theory frame of reference, we can conceptualize this process not only in terms of projection but also in terms of a role reversal, in which unacceptable feelings and motivations (in our example, aggressive wishes to criticize and compete) are consciously represented but are dissociated from the self and attributed to an object representation, while the patient identifies with the object of her now projected impulses. (In our example, the patient identifies with a naive and trusting victim of aggression rather than experiencing herself as someone who harbors aggressive impulses toward someone who is naive and trusting.) As in classical descriptions of neurotic-level projection, the connection between the feelings and motivations that the patient has projected and the corresponding self representation is repressed. What we wish to add is the recognition that not only is the patient ridding herself of certain conflictual motivations, she is also, at the same time, identifying with others (in our example, motivations to naively trust).

SUGGESTED READINGS

Akhtar S: Broken Structures: Severe Personality Disorders and Their Treatment. Northvale, NJ, Jason Aronson, 1992

Kernberg OF: Identity: recent findings and clinical implications. Psychoanal Q 65:969–1004, 2006

Kernberg OF: Projection and projective identification: developmental and clinical aspects, in Aggression in Personality Disorders and Perversions. New Haven, CT, Yale University Press, 1992, pp 159–174

Kernberg OF, Caligor E: A psychoanalytic theory of personality disorders, in Major Theories of Personality Disorder, 2nd Edition. Edited by Clarkin JF, Lenzenweger MF. New York, Guilford Press, 2005, pp 115–156

McWilliams N: Psychoanalytic Diagnosis: Understanding Personality Structure in the Clinical Process. New York, Guilford, 1994

Mischel W, Shoda Y: Integrating dispositions and processing dynamics within a unified theory of personality: the cognitive-affective personality system, in Handbook of Personality: Theory and Research, 2nd Edition. Edited by Pervin LA, John OP. New York, Guilford, 1999, pp 197–218

PDM Task Force: Psychodynamic Diagnostic Manual, Personality Patterns and Disorders. Silver Spring, MD, Alliance of Psychoanalytic Organizations, 2006

Shapiro D: Neurotic Styles. New York, Basic Books, 1965

Vaillant G: The Wisdom of the Ego. Cambridge, MA, Harvard University Press, 1993

Westen D, Gabbard G, Blagov P: Back to the future: personality structure as a context for psychopathology, in Personality and Psychopathology. Edited by Kruger RF, Tackett JL. New York, Guilford, 2006, pp 335–384

Zetzel ER: The so-called good hysteric. Int J Psychoanal 49:256–260, 1968

3

INTERNAL OBJECT RELATIONS, MENTAL ORGANIZATION, AND SUBJECTIVE EXPERIENCE IN PERSONALITY PATHOLOGY

We discuss in this chapter the relationship between internal object relations and personality pathology. As discussed in Chapter 2 ("A Psychodynamic Approach to Personality Pathology"), in higher level personality pathology, identity is consolidated and internal object relations and dominant self experience are relatively well integrated and stable. This structural organization corresponds with a well-developed capacity for self-reflection and a relatively realistic and stable experience of self and significant others. In areas of conflict, however, internal object relations tend to be less well integrated and conflictual representations of self and other are split off from dominant self experience. Further, in areas of conflict the capacity for self-reflection is often to some degree impaired.

In this chapter we make a link between the relatively poorly integrated quality of conflictual object relations and defensive operations, and we describe a variety of ways in which internal object relations are used to serve defensive functions. Dynamic psychotherapy for higher level personality pathology (DPHP) is designed to promote integration of conflictual internal object relations, a process sometimes referred to as *structural change*. We link the progressive integration of internal object relations and structural change in higher level personality pathology to the working through of conflicts characteristic of the "depressive position" (Klein 1935). As depressive conflicts are worked through and ambivalence is tolerated, we see increased integration of internal object relations and decreased personality rigidity.

REPRESENTATIONS OF SELF AND OTHERS AND PERSONALITY RIGIDITY

In our model, unconscious conflicts and defensive operations are embedded in mental life in the form of internalized relationship patterns (Kernberg 1992). As we have described, from a structural perspective, the patient with higher level personality pathology presents with personality rigidity in the setting of identity consolidation. Identity consolidation implies integration of the patient's conscious and preconscious self and object representations to form a stable yet fluid experience of self and of significant others. At the same time, the patient with higher level personality pathology struggles with particular aspects of his conscious and unconscious experience of himself and others that are not compatible with his overall sense of himself and the world. These conflictual experiences of self and other, along with associated affects, are split off from dominant self experience and remain relatively resistant to change or to environmental influence. Defensive operations that keep these object relations out of conscious awareness introduce rigidity into personality functioning, and contexts that activate conflictual representations of self and other will stimulate anxiety.

REPRESENTATIONS OF SELF AND OTHERS AND SUBJECTIVE EXPERIENCE IN PERSONALITY PATHOLOGY

Internal object relations, derived from the past but active in the present, color the experience of internal and external reality. In the patient with higher level personality pathology, the internal object relations closest to consciousness are relatively complex, well integrated, and well differentiated. In everyday life, there is typically a relatively good "fit" between objective, external reality and the patient's subjective experience as represented in the particular internal object relations activated at any given moment. As a result, there is limited distortion of external reality and a relatively sophisticated capacity to accurately perceive the inner experience of others (*empathy*).

In areas of conflict, however, the inner world of the patient with higher level personality pathology is relatively rigid and fixed, and his experience of external reality will be colored and to some degree distorted by his defensive needs. As a result, in areas of conflict, the patient's inner experience will correspond less closely and flexibly with external reality than will his experience in areas that are not conflictual. Further, in areas of conflict, the patient's internal representations of self and other will be less well integrated, less well differentiated, and more extreme than is characteristic of his usual level of integration, and the affects associated with these representations typically will be more intense and threatening.

In sum, in the patient with higher level personality pathology, enactment of *conflictual* internal object relations will often lead to subtle distortion of the patient's experience of himself and of the world and other people. DPHP is designed to promote the emergence of such conflictual self and object representations into consciousness. During the course of treatment, the activation of conflictual object relations and their enactment in the patient's current relationships, including the relationship with the therapist, present the major route of access to the patient's internal world.

The mental organization of the patient with higher level personality pathology can be contrasted with that of the patient with more severe personality pathology, for whom identity is not fully consolidated and representations of self and others are unstable, poorly integrated, and polarized. This internal situation, typical of the severe personality disorders, leads to chronic, gross distortions of the individual's experience of self and others (Kernberg 1984). In contrast to higher level personality pathology, where more primitive or extreme object relations are *repressed*, in more severe personality pathology they are *dissociated* and fully accessible to consciousness. In therapy with patients with severe personality disorders, the activation of these internal object relations leads to rapid distortion of the relationship with the therapist. DPHP is designed to contain acting out while promoting the integration of dissociated self and object representations through interpretation and containment (Clarkin et al. 2006).

SELF-REFLECTION AND PERSONALITY PATHOLOGY

The patient with higher level personality pathology typically enjoys a relatively well developed capacity for self-reflection; thus, when a patient with higher level personality pathology enacts a particular conflictual internal object relation, he is typically at the same time aware of himself doing so. This is because, in the individual with higher level personality pathology, the organized sense of self, corresponding with identity consolidation, functions as an observer or an implicit "third party" in relation to the activation of conflictual internal object relations. In a therapy session, it is the patient's observing self that the therapist talks to and, in essence, joins with. An alliance is formed between the patient's observing self and the therapist in the role of observing the patient with the intention of helping him (Kernberg 2004b).

In contrast, people with severe personality pathology typically have a more limited capacity for self-reflection, especially in the setting of high affect states. When a particular object relation is activated, the individual will often be immediately and entirely involved in the enactment of the dyadic object relation, and subjective experience will lack the self-observing or "triangular" quality that is associated with self-awareness. Consequently, patients with severe personality pathology can have difficulty distinguishing between the therapist as he is experienced in the transference and the therapist in his helping, observing role, especially in the setting of highly charged affect states. As a result, in the patient with a severe personality disorder, the alliance between therapist and patient will be more tenuous and less stable than in the patient with higher level pathology (Bender 2005).

Even though people with higher level personality pathology are generally able to self-reflect, the capacity for self-reflection is weaker in areas of conflict. This is to say that when conflicts are activated and affects become intensified, thinking becomes more concrete and experience more immediate. As thinking becomes more concrete, the capacity to appreciate the symbolic nature of mental representations and to reflect on them can be compromised.[1] In treatment, as unconscious conflicts are activated, the observing therapist will join with the patient's weakened observing self to encourage self-observation and self-reflection. This process, repeated over and over again in each session and throughout the treatment, will help the patient develop a greater capacity for self-reflection, even in the face of anxiety and unconscious conflict. During the course of treatment, as conflicts are worked through, the patient's capacity for self-reflection will deepen and he will rely less heavily on the therapist to facilitate self-exploration.

CLINICAL ILLUSTRATION OF
DEEPENING CAPACITY FOR SELF-REFLECTION

A research scientist came to treatment complaining about problems with self-esteem. Though he was fully able to self-reflect on many aspects of his

---

[1]By *appreciating the symbolic nature of mental representations*, we mean recognizing that thoughts *stand for* things, in contrast to experiencing them *as* things. For example, the thought of a particular dog corresponds to that dog but is not equivalent to the dog itself.

inner world, when it came to his sense of inferiority and defectiveness, his thinking became more concrete. In keeping with this attitude toward himself, early in treatment this man was secretly convinced that he was "the worst patient" in his therapist's practice. In fact, he was so convinced of this that it took him months to share this concern with his therapist. While he could entertain the possibility that it was not true, at the same time he truly believed he must be the most refractory of his therapist's patients. Over time, the patient's therapist invited him to explore the meaning of this view of himself rather than simply to accept it as a material fact. As the patient's conflicts concerning his self-esteem were worked through, he stopped thinking of himself as his therapist's "worst patient."

However, several months later the patient found himself once again experiencing himself in this way. At this point, he held a different attitude toward his self-condemnation than he had had at the beginning of the therapy. He was now able to maintain awareness that what he was thinking and feeling reflected his current mental state rather than a material fact—that he was experiencing a particular self representation, activated at a particular time for a particular reason. This enabled him to reflect on the meaning of the thought, in contrast to experiencing it as a concrete reality as had occurred early on.

THE DEVELOPMENTAL PAST AND PSYCHOTHERAPY OF PERSONALITY PATHOLOGY

The relationship between a patient's historical, developmental past and the internalized object relations activated during the course of psychotherapy is complex. Patients with higher level personality pathology present with an array of conscious, preconscious, and unconscious representations of the self in relation to parents and other important people from past and present life that will be activated during the course of treatment. These representations are often coherent and credible, particularly early in treatment. This is in marked contrast to the situation with patients with severe personality pathology, who typically present with self and object representations that are unstable, polarized, and fantastic.

However, when treating a patient with higher level personality pathology, it is important for the therapist to understand that the patient's conscious views of his relationships with early caretakers and other significant figures do not necessarily correspond to a fixed, historically valid reflection of external reality. Rather, these images of relationships are understood as constructions, compromises between memory (as affected by developmental stage), fantasy, and defense, colored by current circumstances (Kernberg 1992). Further, the patient's current relations with and experiences of others, including the therapist during the course of treatment, are viewed as equally complex and fluid constructions. Over the course of a therapy, the patient will experience a broad array of images of these relationships, some loving and some hateful, some sexual, some nurturing, some relatively mature, and some seemingly more primitive or childlike (Schafer 1985).

OBJECT RELATIONS AND SUBJECTIVE EXPERIENCE IN PERSONALITY PATHOLOGY

In sum, the degree of rigidity versus flexibility of a person's defensive operations, as well as the quality and degree of integration of the internal object relations embedded in his inner life, will determine his subjective experience of inner and outer reality. The normal personality is free to experience a wide array of object relations, activated by internal and external circumstances. The individual with higher level personality pathology, in contrast, must rigidly defend against conscious and unconscious experiences of self and other that are associated with areas of conflict. To do this, the patient maintains a state in which conflictual aspects of self and other are either repressed or dissociated and are not part of his dominant experience. Situations that activate these warded-off object relations will generate anxiety and defensive distortion of internal and external reality.

In DPHP, we use the treatment setting in conjunction with the analysis of resistance to activate conflictual object relations, thereby helping the patient and the therapist gain access to unconscious experiences of self and others and associated defensive operations.

INTERNAL OBJECT RELATIONS AND DEFENSIVE OPERATIONS IN PERSONALITY PATHOLOGY

Our psychotherapeutic technique is centered on the analysis of the internal object relations activated, moment to moment, in the treatment setting. This is because the internal object relations activated by conflictual situations in the patient's current life and in the treatment situation offer a window into the patient's inner world, and, ultimately, into his unconscious life. As the patient's internal object relations come to life in his current relationships—including the relationship with the therapist—the conflictual motivations, defenses, and anxieties underlying personality rigidity and associated symptoms will come to light.

As we have described, in an unconscious conflict, both defenses and conflictual motivations are represented and subjectively experienced as internalized relationship patterns, linked to unconscious fantasies about desired or feared relationships. The representations of self and other serving defensive functions will be relatively accessible to consciousness, while the less well integrated and more highly affectively charged internal object relations associated with the expression of conflictual motivations will be repressed or dissociated.

Through the course of treatment, we expect to uncover and work through core conflicts, beginning with exploration of relationship patterns that are defensively mobilized and moving toward underlying, more highly conflictual object relations. As patient and therapist come to understand the expressive and defensive functions of a given internal object relation, other internalized relationship patterns, previously defended against, will come to light. In this way, as the treatment progresses, patient and therapist develop an increasingly complex and profound understanding of the patient's presenting difficulties and anxieties.

Enactment of a particular object relation can serve defensive functions in a number of ways. First, enactment of a defensive internal object relation can support repression of other, more conflictual internal object relations that are closer to the direct expression of conflictual motivations. This is what we see in *repression proper*. Second, enactment of any internal object relation functions as a compromise formation to the degree that unacceptable motivations are attributed to an object representation while being split off from the paired self representation. This is what we see in *neurotic projection*. Third, enactment of a conflictual object relation can serve a defensive function to the degree that enactment of this object relation remains poorly integrated with dominant self experience. This is what we see in *splitting or dissociation.*

The three defensive processes that we have just outlined all involve distancing conflictual motivations from the self. At the same time, they entail distancing or separating conflictual motivations from other motivations with which they are in conflict. The focus on the relationship between conflictual motivations and self experience is reflected in the *goals* of DPHP. The focus on the relationship between conflictual motivations and other, less conflictual motivations is reflected in the *strategies and tactics* of DPHP and in our underlying model of how the treatment works. We elaborate on these ideas in the pages that follow.

REPRESSION: LAYERING OF INTERNAL OBJECT RELATIONS

The process whereby enactment of internal object relations closest to consciousness defends against awareness or enactment of other, more threatening internal object relations is an example of repression proper. Repression can be thought of in terms of the "layering" of internal object relations. By layering, we refer to the dynamic situation in which those internal object relations at or close to the conscious surface protect against activation of underlying layers of unconscious mental contents. Both defenses and unacceptable motivations are represented as internal object relations that are associated with unconscious fantasies about desired and feared relation-

ships. As a result, when a patient uses repression to defend against unconscious conflict, what we can observe are behaviors that reflect the enactment
of defensive object relations. Enactment of these defensive object relations
functions to maintain repression of conflictual internal object relations that
are more closely tied to the expression of conflictual wishes, needs, and fears.

CLINICAL ILLUSTRATION OF LAYERING OF INTERNAL OBJECT RELATIONS

Consider the young man who is habitually eager to please. This man is enacting an internalized relationship pattern of a pleasing-child self in relation
to an attentive parent. This internal object relation, automatically and routinely activated, serves to avoid awareness of other views of self and other
that are more threatening ("conflictual") and closer to the expression of
conflictual motivations. For example, enactment of the internal object relation of the pleasing-child self and the attentive parent may serve as a defense
against activation of an internal object relation comprising an angry child
and a sadistic parent. At the same time, the activation of this entire conflict,
both defense and impulse, ultimately also functions to defend against activation of other conflicts. For example, if this man were in therapy, it might
turn out that his anxiety about anger and sadism defends against sexual conflicts, perhaps experienced as a relationship between a seductive parent and
an overstimulated child self.

PROJECTION SUPPORTS REPRESSION: ROLE REVERSAL AND INTERNAL OBJECT RELATIONS

Another way in which enactment of an internal object relation can support
repression is by attributing unacceptable motivations to an object representation while repressing the connection between these unacceptable motivations and the self. This defensive operation can be distinguished from
repression proper—what we have referred to as layering—in which a conflictual motivation is entirely banished from consciousness. Instead, a conflictual motivation is banished not entirely from consciousness, but rather
from conscious self experience.

This process involves *projection*, insofar as the conflictual motivation has
been split off or dissociated from self experience and attributed to an object, and *repression*, insofar as the subject has repressed all awareness of the
connection between the self and the unacceptable impulse. In essence, the
patient has split apart conflicting motivations, attributing the more conflictual motivation to an object representation while identifying with the
less conflictual motivations. When this object relation is enacted, the patient will experience his own, projected impulse coming toward himself
from an object while the patient consciously assumes the attitude of the

split object representation. Because the patient's conflictual motivations are experienced as coming from an object and directed toward the patient, while the patient consciously identifies with the object, this defensive operation can be conceptualized as a form of role reversal. Projection can be contrasted with projective identification in that in projection, there is no emotional awareness of the impulse that is projected, nor is there an unconscious induction of the projected impulse in the object (Kernberg 1992).

CLINICAL ILLUSTRATION OF ROLE REVERSAL

Consider the young woman who habitually enacts an internal object relation composed of an innocent, loving, nonsexual self in relation to a sexual and seductive object. In this object relation, all sexual interest and seductiveness is attributed to the object representation, while the self representation has no connection to these impulses. This young woman's conscious self experience is of love and sexual naïveté, perhaps associated with feeling herself in a childlike position. This self experience defends against awareness of her sexual feelings.

We can see that embedded in the object relation is an expression of the patient's sexual interest and her wishes to be seductive, although these are entirely dissociated from the loving, naïve self and experienced as coming from the object. As a result, we can view this internal object relation as both a covert expression of and a defense against the patient's own sexual and seductive impulses. (This is what is meant by the term *compromise formation*.) Even though this young woman is unable to keep her sexual desires entirely out of awareness, she is entirely unaware of her connection to them.

At the beginning of treatment, the patient with higher level personality rigidity will be predominantly identified with one side of a given internalized relationship pattern. By the end of a successful treatment, the patient will come to tolerate awareness of his identification with both sides of the relationship. For example, in the clinical illustration immediately above, the patient was initially identified with the naïve, loving, childlike self representation; during the course of her treatment, she came to tolerate awareness of her identification with her sexual and seductive self as well. From this more tolerant position, she was able to observe the defensive functions served by her identification with each half of the object relation. In essence, identifying with the naïve, loving, child defended against anxieties associated with sexuality, whereas identifying with the sexual figure defended against anxieties associated with vulnerability and love.

One patient will find one position more anxiety provoking; another, the reverse. In the course of treatment we should see the patient's identifications with both sides of the relationship emerge into consciousness, though this will not necessarily happen immediately. As these varied identifications emerge and are worked through, the patient will be free to have a more varied and fluid self experience. For example, the patient who presents with naïveté should be free to enjoy her sexual and seductive impulses, and she should no longer need to separate vulnerability and love from sexuality, leaving her with a greater capacity to experience and enjoy erotic love.

FROM PROJECTION TO INTEGRATION

The defensive operation we have just illustrated is typically conceptualized as a form of projection. In our example, unacceptable sexual needs and wishes, along with aspects of the self tied to erotic motivations, are split off from self experience and projected into an object. In this formulation, the emphasis is on the contents of the patient's projection. However, our clinical example illustrates how this sort of defensive maneuver typically involves not only the projection of unacceptable motivations and associated emotional states, but also the *segregation* of different sets of motivations that are in conflict. In essence, we are suggesting that in projection, we see not only the attribution of a conflictual motivation to an object but also the segregation of two sets of motivations, one of which is conflictual, within an object relation.

To return to our example for a moment, we are suggesting that this patient's problem is not adequately described by the observation that she finds her sexual wishes unacceptable and therefore needs to extrude them. Rather, a more complete description would include the patient's particular difficulty in integrating sexual needs and relationships with dependent needs and relationships; her defensive strategy is not simply to rid herself of unacceptable sexual motivations, but rather to ensure that sexual motivations remain segregated from dependent needs. In the initial configuration, this young woman contains all of the dependent needs that are embedded in her romantic relations within herself, while all sexual needs are contained within the object. She is entirely free of sexuality, while he (the object) is entirely free of dependency needs.

What we are suggesting is that within an object relations theory frame of reference, it can be useful to think less about projection and more about the compartmentalization or segregation, within a single object relation, of motivations that are in conflict. This view is consistent with what we see clinically as a patient's defenses start to become less rigid. Typically, what we see first is a role reversal—a shift from a naïve patient and a sexual object to a sexual patient *in relation to* a naïve object (Kernberg 1992). This is to say that even though the patient is now better able to tolerate awareness of her own sexual needs, it is only safe to do so in a setting in which her sexuality and dependency needs remain segregated. It is only after the working through of the patient's identifications with both sides of the split (the sexual and the dependent), and of the manner in which one identification defends against the other and also defends against the anxiety of simultaneously experiencing two conflicting sets of motivations, that we see increased integration and decreased personality rigidity.

For this patient to become free of sexual and romantic inhibitions, not only will she have to tolerate awareness of her own sexual desire but, in addition, she will have to undo the separation of sexual and dependent motivations and integrate the two of them. This shift would be represented as an internal object relation of a loving, dependent, sexual self in relation to a loving, sexual object. Integrating sexual and dependent impulses in this way is predicated on the patient's coming to terms with the fantasies and anxieties associated with oedipal conflicts.

SPLITTING AND DISSOCIATION IN HIGHER LEVEL PERSONALITY PATHOLOGY

In addition to repression-based defenses, patients with higher level personality pathology also rely on dissociation or splitting-based defenses in the face of unconscious conflict. Splitting and dissociation are in some ways similar to projection, insofar as motivations that are in conflict with one another, along with associated aspects of self experience, are kept apart. However, whereas projection can be conceptualized in terms of segregating motivations within a single object relation, splitting-based defenses can be conceptualized in terms of segregating conflicting motivations between different object relations. And where projection involves repression of the connection between an impulse and the self as well as between two impulses, splitting and dissociation do not involve repression, nor do they entail completely severing the connection between conflictual impulses and the self.

In higher level personality pathology, splitting and dissociation involve separating two motivations that are in conflict, associating each with a different set of internal object relations, and ensuring that there is no connection between the dissociated object relations. In contrast to projection, in splitting and dissociation, nothing is repressed—both sets of object relations are consciously experienced. What we see clinically is that while conflictual motivations are consciously experienced and enacted, they remain at the same time split off from other motivations and aspects of self experience with which they are in conflict. This process avoids the psychological dangers associated with integrating motivations that are in conflict and at the same time ensures that the expression of conflictual motivations is not completely integrated into self experience. Patients frequently dissociate dependency from aggression; love and/or dependency from sexuality; and aggression from love and tenderness.

CLINICAL ILLUSTRATION OF SPLITTING AND DISSOCIATION IN HIGHER LEVEL PERSONALITY PATHOLOGY

To illustrate the impact of dissociation and splitting on internal experience and external functioning in higher level personality pathology, let's return to the clinical example of the young woman with conflicts involving her erotic desires. In our initial discussion of this patient illustrating the use of projection, she experienced herself as a loving, dependent person free of sexual desire, in relation to a sexual person with no dependency needs. In contrast, if this patient were to rely predominantly on splitting rather than projection to address her sexual conflicts, we would see one set of object relations in which she enacts loving and dependent needs and wishes free of erotic overtones, and another, separate, set of object relations in which she enacts erotic excitement and seductiveness. In her external life, the patient would be able to gratify her sexual desires, but only to the degree that she is able to maintain a separation between dependent and erotic object relations.

OEDIPAL CONFLICTS

We have discussed the descriptive and structural features of personality pathology. At this point we turn to the topic of psychodynamics. When we use the term *psychodynamic* or when we discuss a particular patient's "dynamics," we are addressing the nature and developmental origins of the conflicts that are associated with the patient's personality pathology. We can conceptualize the core psychological conflicts commonly encountered in people with higher level personality pathology in terms of two overarching categories of anxieties. The first group of conflicts can be conceptualized in terms of *dyadic* object relations; these conflicts are organized around fears about being vulnerable and depending on and trusting others. The second group of conflicts can be conceptualized in terms of *triadic* object relations; these conflict are often organized around fears about competing with someone to obtain something or someone that both parties desire. Triadic object relations and conflicts are often associated with oedipal dynamics.

TRIANGULAR CONFLICTS AND THE OEDIPUS COMPLEX

The hallmark of oedipal development and conflict is that it is *triadic*, by which we mean that the self's relation to a loved, desired, or needed person is inextricably tied, psychologically, to a third party. The prototype of triadic internal object relations is the relationship between the child and the two parents as a couple. The developmental hurdles of the oedipal situation entail coming to terms with living in a world in which the people we love and need have relationships with others that exclude us. The capacity to appreciate and grapple with this dilemma is predicated on the awareness of a self with a subjective inner life, of another person separate from the self and not controlled by the self, and of a third party. This constellation signifies a relatively mature level of psychic and cognitive development, and it is typically associated with the capacity for self-observation and self-reflection.

In oedipal conflicts, sexual, dependent, competitive, and aggressive wishes, needs, and fears are linked to childhood fantasies of breaking up the parental couple to possess the sole attention of one or both parents, excluding and triumphing over the other parent and/or over other members of the family. As a result, sexual, dependent, competitive, and aggressive needs and wishes, and the fantasies to which they are linked, are conflictual, and enactment of the object relations associated with expression of sexual, dependent, and aggressive motivations will lead to feelings of guilt and loss, coupled with fantasies of feared retribution.

For example, for the oedipal girl, fantasies of possessing father as her own love object will also involve fantasies of displacing, triumphing over, and perhaps doing away with mother. To the extent that the girl retains a positive image of her mother in the face of her rivalrous feelings, she is confronted with a painful conflict. Her wishes to gratify her sexual and sadistic impulses, along with her competitive and narcissistic desires to possess father, are in conflict with her love for mother, her dependency on mother, and her fear of mother's retribution.

In the adult, this conflict can remain unresolved and buried. Situations connected to oedipal conflict, particularly sexual intimacy and competitive struggles, will stimulate anxiety, guilt, and fear. It is because of the unconscious link between sexual love and guilt-provoking childhood fantasies of incestuous triumph that patients with prominent oedipal conflicts have difficulty integrating passionate sexuality with tenderness and love.

DYADIC CONFLICTS AND DEPENDENCY

Although triangular conflicts often prove to be core dynamics in patients with higher level personality pathology, these patients also present to treatment with dyadic conflicts. In contrast to triangular conflicts that involve living in a world in which we depend on others while acknowledging that they have needs of their own and relationships with others that exclude us, dyadic conflicts typically involve the ups and downs of depending on others per se, without attention to third parties. The prototype of the dyadic relationship is the interaction between the young child and its caretaker, and, in particular, the child's experiences of satisfaction and frustration in that relationship. The way in which dyadic conflicts are organized will relate to the individual's capacity to establish trusting, dependent relationships.

Dyadic conflicts are sometimes conceptualized as "preoedipal"—referring to the child in relation to a parent as caretaker, in contrast to the child in relation to the parental couple.

In triangular conflicts, gratification implies taking something from someone else who wants it, and frustration and deprivation are experienced in terms of someone else's getting "something I want." In contrast, in dyadic conflicts, gratification is experienced in terms of getting "something I want" from "someone who will always give me what I want," and frustration and deprivation are experienced in terms of not getting "what I want" from "someone who doesn't want to give me what I want." Because there is no triangulation, all the love stimulated and signified by gratification, as well as all the rage stimulated by frustration, are focused on a single object who is experienced as entirely responsible for whatever happens in the interaction. For example, the young girl's experience with mother generates representations of a beloved mother who feeds and protects the child, as well as contradictory representations of an unavailable or distracted mother who engenders frustration and envy.

Dyadic and triangular conflicts typically are condensed and play off one another. Conflicts involving dependency and trust make it difficult to negotiate triangular conflicts and the oedipal situation; at the same time, experiencing a situation in terms of dyadic needs and conflicts can serve as a way to avoid oedipal-level, triangular anxieties about competition and sexuality. As a result, while the ultimate dynamic focus of DPHP is often a triangular conflict, unresolved conflicts about dependency may take center stage at any phase of the treatment. The activation of dyadic object relations in the treatment will at times be used defensively to avoid oedipal-level conflict, just as the activation of oedipal-level material will be at times used to defend against the emergence of dyadic conflicts involving dependency and trust.

THE DEPRESSIVE POSITION

Sigmund Freud introduced the construct of the Oedipus complex (Freud 1953 [1900]) and ultimately made it the cornerstone of his theory of psychological conflict and pathology. Klein further developed our understanding of the triangular conflicts of oedipal-level conflict by integrating the Oedipus complex into her construct of the *depressive position* (Klein 1935). In the depressive position, the subject begins to tolerate ambivalence, bringing an awareness of hostility toward and from beloved objects. Awareness of ambivalence leads initially to depression, pain, loss, guilt, and remorse and the wish to make reparation. Ultimately, the individual takes responsibility for and mourns the damage he has done to his objects in fantasy as he comes to tolerate emotional awareness of the loss of ideal images of himself and his objects (Segal 1964).

Working through depressive anxieties enables the individual to take responsibility for his own destructive, aggressive, and sexual impulses while tolerating awareness of these impulses in others; to establish mutually dependent relationships; and to feel love and concern for others, who are experienced as separate and complex. Further, the capacity to experience others as separate is closely tied to the capacity for symbolic thought (Spillius 1994).

Klein contrasts the depressive position with the more "primitive" *paranoid schizoid position* (Klein 1946), in which ambivalence is not tolerated, splitting predominates, and positive, loving and negative, aggressive object relations are kept apart. Where the central anxieties of the depressive position have to do with guilt over one's own potential to be destructive or hurtful, anxieties of the paranoid schizoid position are experienced as coming toward, rather than stemming from, the subject, and have to do with fears of annihilation. In the paranoid schizoid position, ego boundaries are relatively porous and objects are controlled; thought is concrete and omnipotent.

Contemporary views of the paranoid schizoid and depressive positions emphasize that these are two ways of organizing psychological experience; the two positions are conceptualized as two different mental states that exist in a more or less stable equilibrium within all of us (Bion 1963; Steiner 1992). Each position is associated with its own set of anxieties and defensive operations. In addition, the two positions imply different degrees of integration of psychological structures; poorly integrated psychological structures and split or "part" objects predominate in the paranoid schizoid position, and better integrated psychological structures and "whole" objects predominate in the depressive position.

The structuring of the patient's defensive organization at a paranoid schizoid or a depressive level differentiates patients with severe personality pathology from patients with higher level personality pathology. This is to say that from a structural perspective, the psychological organization of the paranoid schizoid position corresponds to the internal world of the patient with severe personality pathology, whereas the depressive position corresponds to the organization of the internal world of the patient with higher level personality pathology. From a dynamic perspective, however, the patient with higher level personality pathology moves *between* depressive and paranoid orientations, and the moment-to-moment fluctuations between a paranoid schizoid and a depressive mode of functioning is characteristic of the psychotherapy of these patients. When treatment is successful, we see the repeated and progressive working through of cycles of paranoid and depressive anxieties that enable the patient to make a gradual shift toward a more solidly depressive mode of functioning.

Thus, what we see clinically, at the level of moment-to-moment experience, is that the patient will move between paranoid and depressive ways of organizing his experience. This is to say that in the setting of consolidated identity and an overall depressive level of functioning, the patient with higher level personality pathology will present with a fair amount of variability and fluidity with regard to the degree of integration of his internal objects, the degree to which he is able to take responsibility for his own impulses, the degree to which he experiences guilt and concern rather than paranoia and fear, and the degree to which he is able to maintain a capacity to observe himself and to think symbolically.

From a dynamic perspective, the focus of DPHP primarily involves the working through of paranoid and depressive anxieties stemming from conflicts over sexual, dependent, and aggressive motivations and narcissistic needs. This working through is accomplished by bringing conflicts into consciousness, where conflictual internal object relations can be explored along with the anxieties and defenses associated with enactment of conflictual object relations. As the patient has the opportunity to consciously experience and understand his conflicts as they are activated and enacted in the here and now, and as he is able, progressively, to take responsibility for conflictual motivations, experiencing guilt, loss, and concern, he will work through paranoid and depressive anxieties. In this process, the patient will come to terms with aspects of himself along with aspects of his significant others, past and present, that are painful and/or that are incompatible with his dominant sense of himself and the world.

CLINICAL ILLUSTRATION OF PARANOID AND DEPRESSIVE ANXIETIES IN DPHP

A middle-aged man came to treatment complaining of frustration with his inability to promote himself professionally. In the early weeks of the treatment, the therapist often pointed out to the patient the passive attitude he was assuming in relation to the treatment and in relation to the therapist. In response, the patient felt that the therapist was criticizing him, and he began to worry that the therapist didn't like him. (This initial stance in relation to the therapist on the part of the patient reflected his assuming a predominantly paranoid orientation in the opening phase of the treatment.) There was a somewhat concrete quality to the patient's experience, and he found himself feeling angry at the therapist for not being more supportive and reassuring.

At this point, therapist and patient were able to identify an object relation of a powerful, critical, and rejecting parent in relation to an angry and frightened child, an object relation that had been activated in the transference. The patient was quite struck by this formulation. As he reflected on it, he tearfully remembered a string of painful interactions with his father from early childhood. The patient also reflected on his capacity to have experienced the therapist as so cold and critical when this seemed unwarranted, and toward the end of the session, he wondered out loud what it said about him that he had been so mistrustful of the therapist. (Here we see the patient had shifted to a predominantly depressive orientation.)

When the patient arrived for his next session, the therapist immediately noted a shift in the patient's attitude. The patient was clearly irritated with the therapist and highly critical of any interventions the therapist attempted to make. When the therapist pointed this out, the patient responded that now the therapist must be angry because the patient was being critical of him. (Between the previous session and the current session, the patient had moved away from the depressive anxieties expressed at the end of the previous session to once again assume a paranoid orientation in relation to the therapist.) The therapist thought about what was going on, and then pointed out to the patient that they seemed to be back in the same relationship pattern that they had explored in the previous session, only now with the roles reversed: now the patient was feeling critical and rejecting, while anticipating that the therapist must be angry in return. The therapist also pointed out that in both configurations, the predominant relationship between them was one of hostility.

As the patient considered the therapist's comments, he began to seem less irritable. At this point, the therapist proceeded to remind the patient of the exchange they had had toward the end of the last session. The therapist commented that the things they had talked about had been both poignant and seemingly quite meaningful to the patient at the time, but that at this point, those feelings seemed to have been entirely lost. The patient acknowledged that he had indeed forgotten about the end of the last session. The therapist went on to also remind the patient that he had voiced concern about himself in conjunction with experiencing the therapist as helpful, and the therapist suggested that perhaps the patient's current focus on mutual hostility and criticism served to protect him from some of the more tender feelings he had begun to have at the end of the previous session. (In psychodynamic terms, the therapist was suggesting that the patient had defensively withdrawn from a depressive to a more paranoid orientation, to defend against emerging depressive anxieties; in particular, anxieties associated with feelings of tenderness, vulnerability, and concern.)

STRUCTURAL CHANGE

The ultimate goal of DPHP, that of decreasing personality rigidity, corresponds to changes in the mental organization of the patient. Specifically, decreasing personality rigidity and moving toward a more flexible and adaptive mode of psychological functioning corresponds with progressive integration of psychological structures. The progressive integration of psychological structures is reflected both in the quality of conflictual object relations and in their organization in relation to the dominant sense of self. As psychological conflicts are worked through, we see shifts in the *quality* of conflictual object relations, such that representations become less one-dimensional (more complex and better differentiated) and associated affects become less intense and better differentiated as well. At the same time, we see shifts in the *organization* of conflictual internal object relations such that they coalesce with the nonconflictual self and object representations that comprise the patient's dominant sense of self. These structural changes correspond with an enhanced capacity to emotionally experience and symbolically represent conflictual internal object relations so that they become part of self experience.

INTEGRATION OF INTERNAL OBJECT RELATIONS

From a structural perspective, the working through of psychological conflict results in the assimilation of conflictual object relations into conscious self experience. As part of this process, we can observe a number of related changes in the quality of those object relations closely tied to the expression of conflictual motivations. As conflictual object relations become better *integrated* into conscious self experience, they become more "complex"; by *complexity*, we mean the attribution of more than one motivation to a single object relation or representation. Associated with greater complexity, and with increasing integration, we see changes in the quality of mental representations of self and other such that they become better *differentiated*, by which we mean that they acquire greater subtlety of representation and become more realistic. In addition, as conflictual object relations become better integrated, we see changes in the quality of affective experience associated with enactment of these object relations, such that affects become better differentiated, better modulated, and less overwhelming.

As a result of the integration of conflictual object relations, aggressive motivations and angry feelings, for example, can be represented in the same object relation with loving motivations and tender feelings, and in this process, aggressive impulses become less frightening and less affectively charged. Similarly, sexual wishes can coexist with loving, tender feelings and dependent longings, and in the process can become less threatening and "driven." Integration will mean, for example, that the loving, dependent child can now be critical at times and that the critical, rejecting parent can also feel loving and dependent. Similarly, the loving, dependent child can also have erotic feelings toward his caretaker, and the loving caretaker can tolerate awareness of loving and erotic feelings toward his child, or a single lover can take the place of both "Madonna" and "whore."

As representations of self and other become more complex, less threatening, and less highly affectively charged, they can be assimilated into the mass of representations that comprise the patient's subjective self experience. As a result, changes in the quality of conflictual object relations will also correspond to changes in their relationship to the dominant sense of self. As object relations become better integrated, experiences of self and others that were previously split off can now be tolerated, and they can be assimilated into an overall sense of self and the world able to contain, and flexibly and adaptively manage, pressures for expression of conflictual motivations. The process of progressive integration of conflictual object relations and their assimilation into the dominant sense of self represents a *structural* shift in the patient's mental organization; this is what is meant by *structural change* in DPHP.

CLINICAL ILLUSTRATION OF THERAPEUTIC CHANGE

As an example of the structural and dynamic shifts that we expect to see during the course of a successful therapy, consider the middle-aged, female homemaker who is inhibited about moving into the workplace. Prior to her therapy, in competitive situations she rigidly experienced herself and others as either purely well intentioned or ruthless and worthy of contempt. Further, she consistently needed to avoid, distort, or suck the joy out of experiences that might bring feelings of success or power.

During her therapy, it became clear that in this patient's mind, the specter of competitive success in the professional or sexual arena was associated with an internal object relation of a powerful, ruthless, and triumphant parent interacting with a purely well-intentioned but weak and helpless child self. This internalized relationship pattern was closely connected to a developmental experience that the patient had had with her mother, a successful businesswoman whom the patient had long feared and unconsciously hated. Through her therapy, the patient became aware of competitive and hostile feelings toward her mother, along with an identification with a competitive and hostile maternal object representation, all previously repressed.

With further work, she came to better integrate these representations, and the associated affects of pleasure in triumph, with her representations of the loving parts of herself and her mother. These better integrated representations of success and power could be assimilated into her dominant self experience. As a result, the patient developed the capacity to enjoy the pleasures of competition as she developed a more complex, flexible, and less judgmental image of herself and others in competitive situations.

AMBIVALENCE

Ambivalence can be defined as the capacity to tolerate awareness of conflicting motivations that are simultaneously directed toward the same object. Implicit in what we have described thus far is that the process of integration that constitutes structural change in the higher level personality pathology is predicated on the subject's developing a greater capacity to tolerate ambivalence. Integrated internal object relations are, by definition, ambivalent. Ambivalence implies that the subject is conscious of and able to cope with and integrate aggressive, sexual, exhibitionistic, competitive, self-promoting, loving, and dependent parts of himself and of his objects that are in conflict.

Contemporary Kleinians think of the process of coming to tolerate ambivalence as "working through of the depressive position" (Hinshelwood 1991). This is a construct that is central to contemporary Kleinian approaches to psychopathology and treatment. In the Kleinian model, as in the model of ego psychology, the central dynamic in triangular conflicts is the individual's difficulty tolerating awareness of conflictual aggressive and sexual wishes. However, for Kleinians, the underlying problem is explicitly an inability to fully integrate loving and aggressive motivations (Segal 1964). Aggression toward someone loved is not tolerated. Similarly, to the degree that any sexual relationship is tied to a competitive triumph in a triangle, unconsciously linked to primary objects who are loved and needed, sexual feelings are also not tolerated in a loving and dependent world, and competition becomes problematic.

In the Kleinian model, working through the depressive position entails the subject's emotionally experiencing, and taking full responsibility for, his aggressive and sexual feelings while acknowledging his dependent needs and while staying, psychologically, in a moral world in which love predominates. The central anxiety of the depressive position is the dawning awareness that the subject harbors aggressive motivations toward loved and needed objects who are experienced as autonomous and separate from the self (Segal 1964). As these motivations are no longer dissociated, projected, denied, or repressed, but are instead consciously experienced as part of the self and in terms of wished-for, needed, and feared relationships, the individual can come to take responsibility for his aggression and his wishes to triumph.

This is the first step in the process of integrating previously split-off aggressive and sexual motivations into the loving, tender, and dependent aspects of the experience of self and others. In this process, sexual and aggressive impulses become less threatening, less highly affectively charged, and less concrete; sexual and aggressive wishes and fears, along with the fantasies associated with enacting them, come to be experienced more as thoughts, feelings, desires, and fears, and less as actions that have already been taken. Taking responsibility for destructiveness and wishes for sexual triumph entails tolerating the guilt, remorse, loss, and depression associated with acknowledging one's destructiveness, accepting the realities of triangulation and exclusion, and working through the loss of the hope of an idealized relationship that can be fully protected from aggression and from triangulation. This is the process of *mourning* (Steiner 1996). As part of this process, the subject makes reparation toward those whom he has damaged in fantasy.

Whereas the Kleinian approach emphasizes the difficulty of simultaneously experiencing loving and aggressive feelings toward a single object and integrating conflictual sexual and aggressive object relations into the "ego," or self, we maintain a somewhat broader perspective. We emphasize the difficulties of working through conflicts between love and aggression, but also of integrating each of these motivations with dependent needs, as well as with needs pertaining to the maintenance of feelings of autonomy and self-esteem. In addition, we place greater emphasis on the patient's experience of a relatively well organized and well integrated sense of self, from which conflictual object relations have been split off, with the explicit goal of treatment being to integrate these conflictual object relations into the patient's central, conscious self experience. As a result, the goals of DPHP—to undo dissociation and projection such that conflictual motivations are coherently integrated into the patient's dominant self experience—are similar to, but also to some degree different from, the Kleinian construct of working through the depressive position.

From a dynamic perspective, the goals, strategies, tactics, and techniques of DPHP function to stimulate anxieties pertaining to simultaneously experiencing conflicting motivations within a single object relation, while helping the patient to tolerate, explore, and come to understand these anxieties, and, ultimately, to work them through. In this way, the structural changes brought about by DPHP are also associated with *dynamic* shifts in the patient's mental equilibrium. As part of the process of integration, the patient becomes able to tolerate awareness of conflictual motivations and representations of self and other that were previously repressed or dissociated. These motivations and representations become part of the patient's subjective experience as he develops the capacity to cope with conflictual motivations in a fashion that does not rely on repression, projection, splitting, dissociation, or denial.

As the patient no longer needs to constrict his inner experience to avoid the anxieties associated with activation of conflictual object relations, he can become less rigid and inhibited, and he is free to enjoy a broader range of experiences as his defensive operations become more flexible. This represents a *dynamic* shift in the patient's mental functioning. It is this process of increasing integration of psychological structures—associated with increasing flexibility in mental operations—that moves the patient with personality pathology toward the normal range of functioning during the course of treatment.

SUGGESTED READINGS

Britton R: The Oedipus situation and the depressive position, in Clinical Lectures on Klein and Bion. London, Routledge, 1992, pp 34–45

Greenberg J: Introduction: toward a new Oedipus complex, in Oedipus and Beyond: A Clinical Theory. Cambridge, MA, Harvard University Press, 1991, pp 1–20

Kernberg OF: Object relations theory in clinical practice, in Aggression in Personality Disorders and Perversions. New Haven, CT, Yale University Press, 1992, pp 87–102

Ogden TH: Between the paranoid-schizoid and the depressive positions, in Matrix of the Mind: Object Relations and the Psychoanalytic Dialogue (1986). Northvale, New Jersey, Jason Aronson, 1993, pp 101–129

Ogden TH: The depressive position and the birth of the historical subject, in Matrix of the Mind: Object Relations and the Psychoanalytic Dialogue (1986). Northvale, NJ, Jason Aronson, 1993, pp 67–99

Schafer R: The contemporary Kleinians of London. Psychoanal Q 63:409–432, 1994. Reprinted in Schafer R: Introduction: the contemporary Kleinians of London, in The Contemporary Kleinians of London. Madison, CT, International Universities Press, 1997, pp 1–25

Schafer R: The interpretation of psychic reality, developmental influences, and unconscious communication. J Am Psychoanal Assoc 33:537–554, 1985

Segal H: An Introduction to the Work of Melanie Klein. New York, Basic Books, 1964

Spillius EB: Development in Kleinian thought: overview and personal view. Psychoanalytic Inquiry 14:324–364, 1994

PART **II**

PSYCHOTHERAPEUTIC TREATMENT OF HIGHER LEVEL PERSONALITY PATHOLOGY

THE BASIC ELEMENTS OF DPHP

In the first part of this chapter, we provide an overview of the basic therapeutic tasks of dynamic psychotherapy for higher level personality pathology (DPHP), both to present an overall view of the treatment and to introduce the constructs that will be discussed in detail in the chapters that follow. We next address the topic of *transference*, a construct central to psychodynamic models of treatment. We explain how transference is conceptualized within the framework of object relations theory, and we describe how we have integrated the construct of transference into our object relations–focused approach to psychotherapy. We complete the chapter with a discussion of our model of change—what we hope to see change in our patients as a result of DPHP and how we think the psychotherapeutic technique described in this volume leads to these changes.

THE BASIC TASKS OF DPHP

The first task of the DPHP therapist is to create a setting that will facilitate emergence into consciousness of the conflictual internal object relations underlying the patient's conflicts. The second task is to explore and interpret the anxieties, defenses, and motivations embedded in the conflictual representations of self and other that are affectively dominant in any given session. The third task is to help the patient work through the conflicts that have been interpreted, as they are repeatedly activated and enacted in the patient's current relationships and in his interactions with the therapist. In the process of working through, we emphasize the links between the patient's core conflicts and the treatment goals. The basic tasks of DPHP are summarized in Table 4–1.

TABLE 4–1. The basic tasks of dynamic psychotherapy for higher level personality pathology (DPHP)

Task 1 Bringing conflictual object relations into the treatment

Task 2 Exploring and interpreting unconscious conflicts

Task 3 Working through while emphasizing the treatment goals

BRINGING CONFLICTUAL OBJECT RELATIONS INTO THE TREATMENT

The *treatment setting* refers to the constant features of the treatment. The treatment setting contains the *psychotherapeutic relationship*, a unique relationship established between patient and therapist, designed to promote the activation and exploration of the patient's conflictual object relations. This latter process is facilitated by the *analysis of resistance*. The treatment frame defines the conditions for treatment and the respective roles of therapist and patient in the treatment.

The Treatment Frame

The treatment frame is a defining feature of any kind of psychotherapy and provides the mutually agreed upon structure for the treatment. The treatment frame defines the respective roles of patient and therapist. It also establishes the frequency and duration of sessions, arrangements about handling of scheduling and payment, and expectations about contact, either on the phone or face to face, between patient and therapist outside of regularly scheduled appointments. The treatment frame should be formally established and mutually agreed upon by patient and therapist before treatment begins. The mutual agreement between patient and therapist that establishes the treatment frame is often referred to as the treatment contract (Clarkin et al. 2006; Etchegoyen 1991).

The Psychotherapeutic Relationship

Within the reliable structure provided by the treatment setting, the DPHP therapist and patient establish a special relationship, or object relation, which we refer to as the *psychotherapeutic relationship*. The psychotherapeutic relationship is a highly specialized relationship in which one party, the patient, is encouraged to communicate his inner needs as fully as possible, while the other participant, the therapist, refrains from doing so. The role of the therapist is to use his expertise to broaden and deepen the patient's self-awareness. To this end, the therapist is fully engaged in ongoing efforts to understand the patient's verbal and nonverbal communications and the countertransference. The psychotherapeutic relationship is established by the therapist during the opening phase of the treatment and is the necessary context within which the psychotherapeutic technique described in this book can be implemented.

The Therapeutic Alliance

The *therapeutic alliance* (Bender 2005; Orlinsky et al. 1994) is an important component of the psychotherapeutic relationship. It is the relationship established between the self-observing part of the patient that wants and is able to make use of help and the therapist in his role as helpful expert (Gutheil and Havens 1979). The alliance reflects, on the one hand, the patient's realistic expectation that the therapist has something to offer on the basis of his training, expertise, and concern, and, on the other, the therapist's commitment to help the patient, making use of his developing understanding of him. Most patients with higher level personality pathology are able to establish an alliance relatively easily in the early phases of treatment (Bender 2005; Gibbons et al. 2003; Piper et al. 1991).

Technical Neutrality

As the DPHP therapist establishes a therapeutic alliance with the patient, he maintains what has been referred to as a "neutral" stance (Levy and Interbitzin 1992; Moore and Fine 1995). We stress that technical neutrality does not imply that the therapist is unresponsive or indifferent to the patient's progress. To the contrary, the therapist's attitude toward the patient should reflect an interest in the patient's well-being and a willingness to help, combined with an attitude of warmth and concern (Schafer 1983); when we speak of *technical neutrality*, we refer not to the therapist's attitude toward the patient, but rather to the therapist's attitude toward the patient's conflicts. Technical neutrality calls on the therapist to avoid actively getting involved in or taking sides in the patient's conflicts and to refrain from mak-

ing supportive interventions, such as offering advice or attempting to intervene in the patient's life. Instead, the neutral therapist strives to be as open
as possible to all aspects of the patient's conflicts and behaviors and to maintain a commitment to understanding the patient's inner life as completely
as possible. To this end, the neutral therapist allies himself with the part of
the patient that has a capacity for self-observation (Kernberg 2004b). Technical neutrality is an essential aspect of the DPHP therapist's stance within
the psychotherapeutic relationship.

Support and Supportive Techniques

In psychotherapy, *supportive techniques* are interventions that directly fortify
the patient's adaptive defenses and help him cope with environmental demands. Providing advice, teaching coping skills, supporting reality testing,
and making environmental interventions are examples of supportive techniques. Supportive techniques form the backbone of supportive psychotherapy (see Rockland 1989 for an excellent discussion of psychodynamically
informed supportive psychotherapy) and can be especially helpful to patients with acute and chronic Axis I disorders (American Psychiatric Association 2000).

   In contrast, the DPHP therapist does not routinely make use of supportive techniques. We believe that this approach, though different from
what many others recommend (e.g., Gabbard 2004), is both reasonable and
useful within the therapeutic frame of DPHP. It is reasonable for the
DPHP therapist to abstain from making supportive interventions because
patients with higher level personality pathology generally have sufficient
psychological resources and psychosocial supports to obtain needed emotional and environmental support outside of the therapy and independent
of the therapist. And this approach is useful because abstaining from making supportive interventions enables the DPHP therapist to function more
effectively as an observer of the patient's internal struggles, in contrast to
actively playing a role in them.

   Having said this, we want to make clear the distinction between a patient's feeling emotionally *supported* by a therapist and a therapist's making
use of *supportive techniques*. Even though the DPHP therapist does not typically make use of supportive techniques, patients generally experience
DPHP and the DPHP therapist as extremely supportive; the consistent and
reliable treatment frame, the commitment, interest, and concern of the
therapist, and his accepting and nonjudgmental attitude toward the patient
create an environment that is intrinsically supportive of the patient, of his
inner needs, and of his wish to be understood and to obtain help.

The Therapist as Participant Observer

In DPHP, the therapist maintains a neutral stance when formulating an intervention. However, in his own internal reactions to the patient, rather than striving for neutrality, the therapist makes an effort to open himself up as fully as possible to the patient and to the thoughts and feelings stimulated within him by the patient. The DPHP therapist's ability to maintain a technically neutral stance depends on his capacity to both open himself up to the patient and to observe his interactions with the patient, reflecting upon the private feelings that are stimulated in him by the patient's verbal and nonverbal communications. Thus, the DPHP therapist is both participant and observer (Sullivan 1970), interacting with the patient and allowing the patient to affect him internally, and then standing back and reflecting on what is happening in the session.

Free and Open Communication

In DPHP, the patient's role is to speak in an unstructured way, as freely and openly as possible, about whatever goes through his mind when he is in his therapy session—a process sometimes referred to as *free association* (Moore and Fine 1995). In DPHP, we ask the patient to put aside, temporarily, a specific agenda and instead to allow his mind to wander freely. The rationale for this approach is that it is a highly effective way to bring the patient's conflictual object relations into the treatment, both through the patient's verbal and nonverbal communications and through his *resistances* to open and free communication (Busch 1995; A. Freud 1937).

Analysis of Resistance and Defense

The treatment setting and the therapist's neutrality promote activation of the patient's conflictual object relations. As a result, there is a tendency for the relationship patterns linked to these conflicts to be enacted, as well as an opposing tendency for them to be repressed or otherwise defended against. In treatment, the forces within the patient that defend against enactment of conflictual object relations (i.e., the patient's defensive operations) are activated automatically and are enacted as defensive object relations.

The activation and enactment of the patient's defensive operations in psychotherapy is referred to as "resistance" (Moore and Fine 1995). We use the term *resistance* because, typically, the patient's defensive operations will be manifested as some sort of resistance to open communication or self-observation. The term *resistance* should not be taken to imply that the patient is consciously resisting or intentionally working against the treatment. Resistances, like defensive operations in general, are automatic, largely unconscious, and typically invisible to the patient, even if they are quite apparent to the therapist. *Analysis of resistance* refers to the identification, exploration, and interpretation of the patient's defensive object relations as they are activated and enacted in the treatment.

INTERPRETING UNCONSCIOUS CONFLICT

Interpretations bring to the patient's conscious awareness a conflict that is being activated and either experienced unconsciously, enacted outside the patient's awareness, or expressed in symptoms. Interpretations make connections between defenses, motivations for defense, and the object relations that are being defended against. The process of interpretation will begin from discrepancies or contradictions in what the patient is saying and doing and will lead to explicit hypotheses about the observed discrepancies or contradictions so that sense can be made of them (Kernberg 1984).

The Interpretive Process

Early steps in the interpretive process typically involve clarification and confrontation. *Clarification* entails the therapist's seeking clarification of the patient's subjective experience. Areas of vagueness are addressed until both the patient and the therapist have a clear understanding of what has been said, or until the patient feels puzzled by an underlying contradiction in his thinking that has been brought to light. *Confrontation* involves the therapist's pulling together clarified information, expressed in the patient's verbal and nonverbal communications, that is contradictory or does not fit together, and tactfully presenting the patient with the material that warrants further exploration and understanding. Confrontations implicitly point out activation of the patient's defensive operations and integrate both verbal and nonverbal communications (Etchegoyen 1991).

Interpretation proper follows clarification and confrontation and involves generating a hypothesis about the unconscious conflict that is being defended against. A "complete" interpretation will describe the defense, the anxiety motivating the defense, and the underlying conflictual motivation that is being defended against. However, interpretations are most often offered to the patient in smaller pieces, in stepwise fashion; interpretation is best thought of as a process, beginning with clarification and confrontation, moving on to identification of defensive object relations, followed by exploration of the anxieties motivating defense, and ultimately coming to exploration of the underlying conflictual object relations that have been defended against.

Transference Interpretation

In DPHP, interpretations are made predominantly in the here and now, focusing on what Joseph Sandler (1987) has referred to as the "present unconscious." This means that most interpretations focus on the patient's current anxieties as they are presently activated in his daily life and in the treatment. Sometimes conflictual object relations will be enacted and interpreted in relation to the patient's current interpersonal relationships. At other times, the patient's internal object relations may be enacted and interpreted in relation to the therapist. In the latter case, the interpretation the therapist makes will be a *transference interpretation*. Sometimes conflictual object relations will be simultaneously enacted in the patient's interpersonal life and in the transference. This situation provides the therapist with an opportunity to interpret the link between the patient's conflictual internal object relations, his current difficulties, and the transference.

"Genetic" Interpretation

When treating patients with higher level personality pathology, it is often easy to link conflicts currently active in the therapy to important relationships and events in the patient's developmental past. Interpretations of this kind, that make links to the patient's early history, are sometimes referred to as *genetic interpretations*. Early or excessive focus on linking current conflicts to the patient's past is generally to be avoided, because it can lend an overly intellectualized quality to sessions and will protect the patient from experiencing conflicts in an immediate and affectively meaningful fashion. In contrast, during the later phases of treatment, interpretations that make connections between the patient's early history and his current difficulties and conflicts can work to further deepen the patient's emotional experience of conflictual object relations that have already been interpreted and to some degree worked through.

Insight

An interpretation helps a patient become aware of and make sense of some aspect of his inner life that he has been keeping out of awareness. Because in DPHP we always interpret conflicts that are currently being enacted or are actively being defended against, interpretations help the patient make sense of something that he is actively experiencing (or trying not to experience) in the moment. It is this combination of emotional experience and intellectual understanding (Moore and Fine 1995), in the setting of concern regarding what is newly understood, that we refer to as *insight*. Insight, while often helpful to patients, providing feelings of relief or self-understanding, does not automatically bring about the structural and dynamic changes that are the goals of DPHP. It is the process of *working through* that translates insight into personality change.

Containment

The term *containment* was introduced by Wilfred Bion (1962a). In a general sense, containment refers to the capacity of thinking to temper affect states (Bion 1959, 1962a, 1962b). Containment implies that one can fully experience an emotion without being controlled by that experience or having to turn immediately to action; containment implies both emotional freedom and self-awareness. In DPHP, the therapist contains his own emotional reactions to the patient and to the transference, and in this process he helps the patient to better contain the anxieties activated in the treatment. We believe that, like interpretation, containment on the part of the therapist carries therapeutic potential and is an essential element both in the development of insight and in the process of working through.

In contrast to interpretation, which is an explicit process, containment is an implicit component of the interaction between the patient and the therapist as they explore and come to understand the patient's inner world. In DPHP, the therapist helps the patient put highly affectively charged psychological experiences into words and helps him to reflect on them. The "containing" therapist emotionally responds—internally—to his interactions with the patient and then reflects on whatever the patient is communicating both verbally and nonverbally. In his response to the patient's communication—be it in the form of a verbal or nonverbal intervention—the therapist helps the patient to contain the anxieties stimulated in the therapy. The therapist accomplishes this by communicating that he is accurately registering what the patient is feeling and communicating while, at the same time, he is maintaining a capacity to observe and reflect on his own and the patient's inner states (Bion 1962b; Fonagy and Target 2003; Kernberg 2004b).

WORKING THROUGH AND THE PROCESS OF CHANGE

The process of working through involves the repeated activation, enactment, containment, and interpretation of a particular conflict in a variety of different contexts and over the course of time (Fenichel 1941; Sandler et al. 1992). In fact, the bulk of the work in DPHP involves the process of working through; once core conflicts and associated object relations have been identified, they are repeatedly enacted and explored throughout the course of the treatment. This process of repeatedly activating, enacting, and interpreting a given conflict, and linking the various object relations associated with it, will help the patient gain a deeper and more emotionally meaningful understanding of himself. Further, we believe, it is the process of working through that provides the link between insight and therapeutic change.

Working through relies on the therapist's capacity to contain the anxieties activated in the transference-countertransference, and also on the patient's developing capacity to contain and emotionally experience the anxieties associated with activation of conflictual object relations and associated mental states. In this process, the patient will come to appreciate the role of his identifications with both halves of any particular object relation, as well as the ways that activation of a particular internal object relation or conflict supports repression of others. Ultimately, the patient will come to take responsibility for and tolerate emotional awareness of previously repressed and dissociated aspects of himself and of his internal objects.

In the process of working through in DPHP, we focus on the patient's predominant areas of difficulty, as identified in the presenting complaints and treatment goals. This means that while the patient is encouraged to allow his mind to wander freely without attention to treatment goals, the therapist keeps the treatment goals in mind. As conflictual object relations are enacted in the treatment and the patient's core conflicts come into focus, the therapist will be asking himself, "What is the relationship between the object relations currently being explored and the treatment goals?" In the process of working through, the therapist will focus his interpretations on the relationship between the conflicts currently being enacted and the mutually agreed upon treatment goals, addressing personality rigidity in localized areas of maladaptive functioning while leaving areas of relatively unimpaired functioning undisturbed.

WHAT IS TRANSFERENCE, AND WHAT ROLE DOES IT PLAY IN DPHP?

The term *transference* has a long and complex history (for contemporary views, see Etchegoyen 1991; Harris 2005; Joseph 1987; and Smith 2003). We believe that the term can be defined in a meaningful way only within the framework of a particular model of the mind and treatment.

TRANSFERENCE AND INTERNAL OBJECT RELATIONS

Within the object relational frame of reference used in this book, the term *transference* refers to the playing out, in the present, of patterns of interaction derived from significant relationships in the past. These patterns of interaction reflect the activation of the patient's internal object relations in relation to a person in his current life. In particular, pathogenic experiences and relationships from the past that have profoundly influenced personality structure, along with defenses mobilized in relation to these experiences, tend to be enacted in current interpersonal relationships and to dominate transference developments as well (Kernberg 1992).

In our model, early, significant, and emotionally charged interactions, as well as associated fantasies and defenses, come to be organized in the mind in the form of memory structures or internalized relationship patterns that we refer to as *internal object relations.* These psychological structures function as latent schemas—ways in which the individual can potentially organize his experience—that will be activated in particular contexts (Kernberg and Caligor 2005). Once activated, internal object relations will color the individual's subjective experience and will lead him to act and feel in ways that correspond to the internal object relations currently activated. We think of this process in terms of the individual's "enacting" or "living out" his internal object relations in his daily life. When internal object relations are enacted, psychological structures are actualized. It is this process that we refer to when we use the term *transference.*

The term *transference* is most commonly reserved for occasions when the patient's internal object relations are actualized in relation to the therapist. The term can also be used more broadly to refer to the enactment of the patient's internal object relations in his interactions with another person, without limiting this to the person of the therapist. When used in this way, transference refers to the general process wherein internal object relations, especially conflictual object relations, tend to be actualized or defensively externalized in interpersonal relationships. From this perspective, the transference to the therapist is just a special case of a more general phenomenon in which psychological structures are actualized, or "enacted," in interpersonal life. For purposes of clarity, we will restrict our use of the term *transference* to the more specific meaning of the term, referring to object relations that are enacted in relation to the therapist.

Westen and Gabbard (2002) have approached the construct of transference from the perspective of neuroscience. These authors have suggested that mental representations and internal object relations are encoded at the level of the brain in the form of "associational neural networks." These are networks of neurons that are organized in relation to one another and in relation to other neural structures so that the neurons in a particular associational network will be activated readily, predictably, and simultaneously in response to a particular set of stimuli. In this model, which is both similar to and compatible with our own, representations and transferences exist as potentials that are distributed throughout a network of neural units that are simultaneously activated to produce the representation (Gabbard 2001).

Transference Enactment

In this volume, we use the terms *enact* and *enactment* to refer to the way an individual "lives out" or brings to life his internal object relations in his in- terpersonal life. The term *enact* used in this way describes the process whereby internal object relations, which are latent schemas or potential ways of organizing experience, are actualized as thoughts, feelings, and ac- tions. When we use "enact" in this way, we are speaking from the perspec- tive of the patient. This use of the term is somewhat different from the way the terms *transference enactment* and *transference-countertransference enact- ment* are often used in the psychoanalytic literature.

In the psychoanalytic literature, the term *transference enactment* draws at- tention not only to the patient's experience and behavior, but also to those of the therapist (Moore and Fine 1995). Specifically, transference enactment implies that the therapist's behavior reflects his active participation in play- ing out the transference in his interactions with the patient. Thus, when an- alysts speak of "transference enactment" (i.e., as distinguished from just plain "transference"), it is to emphasize the ways in which the therapist is an active participant in playing out the patient's transference (Steiner 2006).

The distinction between the current psychoanalytic usage of *transfer- ence enactment* and the somewhat different way in which we have been using the term *enactment* calls attention to an area of ambiguity with regard to the degree to which the DPHP therapist actively participates in enacting the patient's transference. From our perspective, when a patient enacts an in- ternal object relation, that internal object relation is "lived" by the patient, regardless of the degree or nature of participation of the other person. For example, if a man is characterologically submissive, from our perspective he is enacting a particular object relation, regardless of how those he is sub- mitting to respond. At the same time, the person to whom he is submitting will always have some sort of a reaction, so that enactment will always in- volve the behavior of both parties.

From this perspective, DPHP is characterized by a steady flow of en- actments in the same way that all interpersonal interactions are. This seems relatively straightforward. However, when we consider the dynamics of en- actment in the setting of the psychotherapeutic relationship, the degree to which the neutral therapist does or does not actively participate in playing out the patient's inner needs and his defensive object relations becomes an important consideration.

The aim of the psychotherapeutic relationship is to create an optimal set- ting within which to explore and understand the patient's inner life. This aim is predicated on the therapist's being emotionally available and responsive to the patient. Further, the patient and the therapist are constantly interacting, so that unless the therapist is a robot, it is not possible—nor is it desirable—to avoid transference-countertransference enactments. At the same time, we believe that when the therapist restrains his own natural inclinations to play out whatever the patient is "pulling for" and maintains a more neutral stance, this will tend to highlight the patient's need to enact particular object relations, making it easier to identify and explore these object relations in the treatment; when the therapist does not actively actualize the patient's transferential expectations, the patient is more likely to become aware that he has expectations of the therapist with regard to his behaving in a certain way.

In DPHP, the therapist deals with the tension between being emotionally available and maintaining neutrality by behaving in a responsive but restrained fashion in relation to the patient, while paying careful attention to the countertransference. This is an attitude that Joseph Sandler (1976) has described as "role-responsiveness." Sometimes the therapist will become aware of a temptation to interact with the patient in a particular fashion before acting on it. At other times, the therapist will only notice his own tendency to interact with a patient in a particular way after the fact. In either case, the therapist can use his reflections on his interactions with the patient to better understand what is going on in the treatment and to formulate a description of the object relations being enacted in the transference.

Enactment and Acting Out

Transference enactment implies that the patient plays out the object relations activated in the transference, regardless of whether or not he is aware of doing so. In contrast, we use the term *acting out* to refer to the situation in which the patient turns to action not to play out conflictual object relations activated in relation to the therapist, but rather to block emotional awareness of them. In this process, the patient avoids whatever discomfort is associated with the underlying conflict. When acting out is used as a general defensive operation, the patient turns to action to make painful affects associated with psychological conflict disappear. When we use the term *acting out* in the treatment setting, it implies the patient turns to action not simply to make painful affects disappear but also as an alternative to the reflective exploration of painful affects in the treatment (Etchegoyen 1991).

For example, if a patient's sexual feelings for her male therapist are expressed in a subtly flirtatious exchange around scheduling, we think in terms of enactment. In contrast, if the patient is unaware of or denies having erotic feelings toward the therapist but finds reason to skip her next session, she is acting out. In the case of acting out, rather than playing out and exploring her erotic feelings, the patient acts as if she can make her erotic feelings for the therapist disappear by ensuring that she does not have face-to-face contact with him.

If this same patient leaves her therapy session, returns to work, and flirts with her boss, with no awareness that her behavior has anything to do with her therapist and no acknowledgement of the conflictual nature of flirting with a man in a position of authority, we might say that she is both acting out in relation to her sexual feelings for her therapist and enacting them. This last example illustrates that acting out and enactment are distinct only in theory. In practice, acting out often involves some degree of enactment, and, at some level, enactment often involves simultaneously both playing out an object relation and trying to avoid making emotional contact with it.

We think of acting out, transference enactment, and transference thoughts as existing on a continuum. At one extreme, in pure acting out, the patient's behavior obscures the object relation activated in the treatment and avoids the affects associated with a particular conflict, as in the case of the patient who cancels a session rather than making emotional contact with the therapist or playing out erotic feelings toward him. In the middle of the continuum, in enactment, object relations activated in the treatment are played out in behavior, and in this way they are brought to the level of emotional experience—but often, at least initially, without self-awareness. Further along the continuum we can see enactments in which the patient is consciously experiencing the object relations that are being enacted in the treatment, or in which the patient is subtly enacting the object relations emerging in his free associations and verbal communication. And finally, at the far end of the continuum, we see transference thoughts, in which object relations activated in the treatment are expressed in thoughts—for example, in the form of a free association, memory, or fantasy—but are not apparently enacted.

The Centrality of Transference in DPHP

In DPHP, we facilitate the activation of the patient's conflictual internal object relations in the treatment. In contrast to psychoanalytic treatment, where emphasis is placed on exploring the patient's internal object relations as they are enacted in relation to the analyst, in DPHP the degree to which the patient "works in the transference" is fairly variable. What we observe is that some patients readily experience their internal object relations in relation to the therapist, while others are highly defended against doing so. In the case of the first group of patients, analysis of the patient's conflictual object relations can take place to a significant degree in terms of the patient's transference to the therapist. In the case of the second group of patients, the same analysis will be made predominantly in terms of the patient's interactions with other people in his life. The difference between the two groups of patients is the degree to which the conflictual internal object relations can be experienced and explored in relation to the therapist and to what extent this experience is defended against.

In the case of the patient who readily enacts such conflicts in relation to the therapist, we are analyzing the patient's transference to the therapist, while in the second case, we are analyzing the patient's "transferences" to the other people in his life, along with his defenses against experiencing these transferences in relation to the therapist. Commonly, analysis of the object relations enacted in external relationships paves the way for exploring the same object relations when the patient enacts them in relation to the therapist later in the treatment. At any given moment, the therapist will decide whether to focus on the transference or on relationships outside the transference on the basis of which material is affectively dominant.

The transference to the therapist is not qualitatively different from the transferences the patient experiences in relation to people other than the therapist. However, in the patient's daily life, his transferential expectations of others will typically be neutralized by the socially appropriate responses of the people around him. In contrast, in DPHP, the patient's transferences to the therapist will be both highlighted and intensified as a result of the therapist's maintaining a neutral stance.

Thus, transferences to the therapist are of particular interest in DPHP because these enactments enable the therapist to experience and explore the patient's conflicts with an immediacy, intensity, and clarity that is lacking when conflicts are explored elsewhere. In addition, we believe that "working through in the transference," a process in which the therapist functions as both a participant and an observer, is an important component of the therapeutic process in DPHP. There is no question that people other than the therapist function as transference objects for the patient, and that effective therapeutic work can by done by analyzing the patient's relationship patterns as they are played out with the important people in his life. However, the therapist's neutrality, in conjunction with his capacity to simultaneously open himself up to the patient while containing his reactions and reflecting on them, distinguishes the transferential relationship with the therapist from other relationships the patient may have.

Transference Developments in Higher Level Personality Pathology

At the core of contemporary views of transference lies the notion of the patient's reliving, or living out in the present, patterns of interaction derived from significant relationships in the past. Thus, in DPHP, the patient will have the experience of his internal object relations literally coming alive in his interpersonal interactions with the therapist and with others in his current life. In DPHP, subjective awareness of transference typically does not emerge as an intellectual abstraction, but rather as an actual experience in which transferential representations of self and other, to a greater or lesser degree, come to dominate the patient's experience of the interpersonal present.

Sometimes, transference developments will emerge in the form of thoughts and/or feelings the patient has during his session, either in relation to the therapist or, initially, in relation to other people in his life. At other times, transferences will be enacted by the patient without the patient's being aware that he is doing so. Here we are talking about identifying the object relations embedded in the patient's behavior—for example, in the tone in which he speaks, in his attitude toward the therapist and toward his own communications, in his body language, or in the "atmosphere" of the session. As a result, when assessing what is going on "in the transference," the therapist will pay attention not only to the contents of the patient's verbal communications and free associations, but also to the patient's nonverbal communications and the countertransference. We are suggesting that the therapist should think not only in terms of "What is the patient communicating to me at this moment?" but also "What is the patient doing with me at this moment?"

Patients with higher level personality pathology tend to develop transferences slowly, gradually, and relatively systematically. The stable and relatively adaptive character defenses that are the hallmark of higher level personality pathology leave the individual quite effectively defended against the emergence into consciousness of repressed and dissociated internal object relations, either in relation to the therapist or in relation to others in the patient's life. Further, because these individuals are able to sensitively and accurately "read" others, they constantly and automatically use subtle interpersonal cues to correct defensive distortions in their interpersonal interactions. In daily life, the individual with higher level personality pathology uses his psychological assets to effectively limit the degree to which his interpersonal interactions are distorted by his unconscious conflicts, and he will do the same thing in the treatment setting.

In the early phases of treatment, transference developments reflect the activation of the patient's character defenses in treatment. Internal object relations more closely tied to underlying conflictual motivations are activated over time, as the treatment progresses and defensive object relations are explored and interpreted. In the treatment of patients with higher level personality pathology, transferences tend to be relatively stable, and one or two transference paradigms will typically dominate the clinical material at any given point in the treatment. Most often, the patient will be consistently identified with a self representation (often a childlike self) over an extended period of time, while attributing to the therapist the corresponding object representation.

In sum, in the psychotherapeutic setting, the patient with higher level personality pathology is relatively well defended against the emergence of his unconscious internal object relations, either in relation to the therapist or in relation to other people in the patient's life. When aspects of the patient's conflictual object relations are activated in the transference, the effects are usually relatively subtle and are easily rationalized by the patient. As a result, in psychotherapy it is necessary to take specific steps to facilitate the emergence and exploration of the patient's conflictual internal object relations in the treatment. In particular, when treating patients with higher level personality pathology we rely on the twice-weekly frequency of sessions, the atmosphere of safety provided by the treatment setting, technical neutrality, and the analysis of resistance to promote the enactment of the patient's internal object relations in the treatment.

MECHANISMS OF CHANGE AND THEORY OF TECHNIQUE IN DPHP

Before moving ahead to a detailed description of psychotherapeutic technique, we will briefly review in schematic form material we have covered thus far pertaining to our model of personality pathology and the goals of DPHP. In addition, we will at this point present our current hypotheses about mechanisms of change in DPHP.

GOALS OF TREATMENT

- The overall goal of DPHP is to increase flexible and adaptive mental functioning and responses to internal and external sources of anxiety, that is, to decrease personality rigidity, in focal areas of functioning in higher level personality pathology.
- Structurally, this shift corresponds to the integration of split-off (repressed and/or dissociated), conflictual aspects of inner life into the patient's dominant self experience.

MODEL OF MENTAL ORGANIZATION

- Patients with higher level personality pathology have a relatively well consolidated and stable conscious self experience that accommodates a variety of affective states, motives, wishes and fears; however, aspects of subjective experience that are conflictual are split off from the individual's conscious sense of self and remain either repressed or dissociated.

- In areas of conflict, psychological experience is more concrete, is more highly affectively charged, and is not as well integrated/is less ambivalent than is mental experience in nonconflictual areas of functioning.
- In the model we are using, psychological conflicts—anxieties, defenses, and conflictual motivations—are represented as clusters of wished-for, feared, or needed internal object relations and associated fantasies, which may be conscious, preconscious, or unconscious.
- Enactment of defensive object relations supports repression and/or dissociation of conflictual motivations and associated anxieties.
- In this model, personality rigidity reflects the habitual enactment of defensive object relations to maintain a psychological situation in which conflictual motivations are excluded from conscious self experience, remaining either repressed or dissociated from the dominant sense of self.

STRUCTURAL CHANGE

- As conflicts are worked through, we see a move from rigidity to more flexible and adaptive functioning in areas of conflict. This shift corresponds to changes in the characteristics of conflictual object relations and in their relation to subjective experience and the dominant sense of self.
- Specifically, as conflicts are worked through, conflictual internal object relations become less concrete (i.e., are experienced consciously as thoughts, feelings, wishes, fears), less highly affectively charged, and more complex (i.e., representations of self and others are associated with more than one motivation, reflecting increased capacity to tolerate ambivalence in areas of conflict), and representations become more highly differentiated, with greater subtlety of representation.
- These changes correspond to the gradual assimilation of conflictual object relations and associated affective experience into conscious self experience, such that conflictual object relations are now comfortably contained within an overall sense of a decent and responsible self living in a predominantly decent but complex world.

DYNAMICS OF CHANGE

- Conflictual object relations and associated affects become accessible to consciousness (conflictual object relations are often first enacted in projected, or inverted, form).

- Conflictual object relations are understood to be part of the self (i.e., are no longer projected, dissociated or denied), and also to reflect identifications with early object ties.
- The patient accepts the loss of ideal images of himself and of his objects.
- Losses are mourned and guilt is worked through.
- The patient comes to tolerate ambivalence in areas of conflict and develops a deepening capacity for concern (in contrast to guilt) for his objects and for himself.

OVERALL PROCESS OF TREATMENT

Schematically, the overall process of the treatment can be conceptualized in terms of two broad steps:

- STEP 1—Undoing repression and dissociation: Conflictual object relations and associated affects emerge into conscious self experience.
- STEP 2—Working through /The process of mourning: The patient tolerates awareness of conflictual object relations, explores associated anxieties and fantasies, works through guilt and loss, and makes reparation. This process enables the patient to better tolerate ambivalence in areas of conflict.

THEORY OF TECHNIQUE AND MECHANISMS OF CHANGE

Using this model, our "theory of technique," which we will review in detail in the chapters that follow, must account for how the technique of DPHP accomplishes the following objectives:

- Helps the patient become conscious of repressed and dissociated, conflictual internal object relations.
- Helps the patient take responsibility for aspects of his inner experience that he has repressed, projected, dissociated, or denied.
- Helps the patient tolerate and mourn the loss of ideal images of self and other.
- Leads to modification of painful, previously repressed or dissociated object relations, so that they can be fully experienced, consciously tolerated, and assimilated into the patient's self experience.

MECHANISMS OF CHANGE: INTERPRETATION AND CONTAINMENT

Our theory of "mechanisms of change" must account for how psychotherapeutic technique accomplishes the aims we have just outlined. Here we are asking:

What is it that the DPHP therapist does with and provides for the patient that makes it possible for him to tolerate awareness of, and take responsibility for, aspects of his inner life that feel intolerable, and to assimilate these intolerable motives and fantasies into his overall sense of himself and his significant others?

It is by now widely acknowledged that there are multiple ways in which psychodynamic psychotherapies facilitate change, and it is also generally accepted that different therapeutic elements work synergistically (Gabbard and Westen 2003). Most contemporary models of change in psychodynamic treatment emphasize the importance of the relationship between therapist and patient as an essential therapeutic element as well as the value of self-understanding in facilitating change (Gabbard 2004).

In our approach to the question of therapeutic change, we also emphasize the central and reciprocal roles played by both the patient's relationship with the therapist and the patient's understanding of himself. We organize our discussion around the constructs of "containment" and "interpretation." Containment is a process embedded in the relationship between patient and therapist. Interpretation is a process that deepens the patient's self-understanding. However, even though we divide our discussion of therapeutic change into two discrete mechanisms of action, containment and interpretation are distinguishable only in theory. In practice, both processes are going on simultaneously and often serve to reinforce one another. A helpful interpretation will often serve a containing function as well as providing insight; similarly, interventions leading up to interpretation often reduce anxiety by way of containment, creating a setting in which a patient is open to hearing and making use of the interpretation that follows.

Furthermore, moving from consideration of the therapist's participation to that of the patient, we can see that the patient's capacity for making use of an interpretation and developing insight is predicated on his developing capacity to contain aspects of psychological experience that he was previously unable to contain. Therefore, the patient's developing capacity to contain conflictual motivations and object relations in focal areas of functioning is a goal of DPHP. In fact, we suggest that *the capacity to contain conflictual object relations, to experience them fully without being controlled by them, is the subjective correlate of the structural ("integration") and dynamic ("flexible adaptation") goals of DPHP.*

It is our hypothesis that it is the combination of containment and insight that makes for psychotherapeutic change. Interpretation without containment typically leads to intellectual discussion of psychodynamics, often without significantly reducing personality rigidity. On the other hand, containment without interpretation and insight leaves the patient dependent on the therapist as an external object; we believe that interpretation *and* insight are both crucial components of the process of working through, allowing the patient to make gains that are retained and will continue to develop after treatment ends (Sandell et al. 2000).

MECHANISM 1: CONTAINMENT

- *Cognitive containment of affect:* Clarification and confrontation put words to more threatening aspects of the patient's psychological experience, helping to cognitively contain the relatively threatening and intense affects associated with conflictual object relations.
- *The containing function of the neutral, tolerant therapist:* The therapist "metabolizes" the patient's projections. By this, we mean that the therapist allows the patient to affect him internally while restraining himself from acting on the patient's projections, and then reflects on the interaction, taking responsibility for his own impulses. What emerges in the therapist's mind is a better integrated, less highly affectively charged, less threatening, and more reflective version of the object relations projected by the patient, which the therapist communicates to the patient. This form of containment takes place both verbally, via interpretation, and nonverbally, by way of the containing functions of the treatment setting and the psychotherapeutic relationship.
- *The containing function of interpretation:* Conflictual motivations and associated anxieties are relatively concrete—it is as if consciously experiencing a desire or conflictual motivation is equivalent to acting on it, and therefore to experience desire is in and of itself tremendously threatening. Further, the subject tends to experience conflictual motivations with an immediacy that leaves him less able than he might otherwise be to observe himself and reflect on his feelings. Similarly, unconscious anxieties also have a concrete quality. (The outcome is experience of the sort expressed by statements like "I am bad by virtue of what I am thinking or feeling" and "You are angry and disapproving.") As conflictual motivations and associated anxieties become conscious, are described and explored in words, and ultimately are interpreted in terms of meanings and functions and underlying fantasies, they become thoughts and feelings rather than concrete "things." That is, they become more clearly "symbolic" aspects of inner experience that can be observed by the patient (and thus can become "triangular").
- *The containing function of transference interpretation:* Conflictual object relations and associated anxieties are often projected, so that the therapist in the transference comes to embody what the patient fears in himself. Putting the patient's transferential experience of the therapist into words in the

form of "therapist-centered interpretations" (Steiner 1994) provides a special form of containment, by implicitly communicating that the therapist can tolerate being and feeling what the patient cannot tolerate in himself.

- *Containment as a facilitator of insight:* As a result of the analyst's containment of the patient's projections, the subjective experiences associated with activation of conflictual object relations become less overwhelming, less concrete, and less threatening; in this way, containment makes it possible for the patient to develop insight, which entails consciously tolerating, cognitively representing, and ultimately taking responsibility for parts of the self that were previously repressed, projected, dissociated, or denied.

MECHANISM 2: INTERPRETATION[1]

- *Paying attention:* Clarification and confrontation call attention to aspects of conscious experience that have been dissociated, ignored, or denied.
- *The interpretation of defensive operations, leading to ego dystonicity:* Identification and exploration of habitual modes of functioning provide a new perspective on personality traits and character defenses; defenses become visible to the patient and ultimately ego-dystonic.
- *The patient's identification with the therapist's observing ego:* The therapist's interventions reflect and convey his capacity to observe and reflect upon the interactions between therapist and patient. The patient's identification with this capacity of the therapist strengthens the patient's observing ego and enhances the patient's capacity to reflect on his inner experience in areas of conflict.
- *The power of the "light of day":* Conflictual object relations and associated anxieties and fantasies, often derived from early childhood, are split off from the adult's conscious self experience; as conflictual object relations and associated fantasies become the focus of conscious attention and are described, explored, and understood from an adult, current-day perspective, they become less threatening.
- *Interpretation supporting symbolization:* As described above, when anxieties are interpreted and understood by the patient in terms of meanings, functions, and origins, they become less concrete and are ultimately viewed as thoughts—representations of mental experience—rather than as material reality.

---

[1] We use the term *interpretation* here to refer to the entire interpretive process, including clarification, confrontation, and interpretation proper.

TABLE 4–2. The therapeutic process in DPHP

Therapist	Patient
Establishing treatment frame	
Establishing psychotherapeutic relationship and technical neutrality	
Observing and reflecting on the patient's psychological experience	Developing treatment alliance
Putting the patient's subjective experience into words	Enhanced capacity for self-observation and self-reflection
Making use of countertransference	
Analyzing resistance to free and open communication	Developing capacity for free and open communication
	Activation and enactment of character defenses and underlying anxieties in the treatment
Containment of anxieties and affect states stimulated in the treatment	
Identification and exploration of defensive object relations	Character defenses become ego dystonic and underlying anxieties emerge into consciousness
Ongoing containment in the setting of exploration and interpretation of anxieties activated in the treatment	Affect states connected to anxieties and conflictual motivations are modified by the therapist's containing and metabolizing rather than actualizing the patient's anxieties and projections
Interpretation of unconscious conflict	
Identification and exploration of conflictual motivations activated in the treatment	
	Affect states connected to anxieties and conflictual motivations are contained by cognitive elaboration
	Enhanced capacity to appreciate the symbolic nature of psychological experience in areas of conflict

TABLE 4-2. The therapeutic process in DPHP *(continued)*

Therapist	Patient
Repeated interpretation and working through	
	Affect states connected to anxieties and conflictual motivations are modified by interpretation and insight as unconscious anxieties and wishes are understood
	Interpretation of defenses and underlying object relations facilitates deepening understanding of psychological experience as symbolic, making it easier to tolerate awareness of and take responsibility for conflictual object relations
	Patient is able to take responsibility for his conflictual motivations, work through guilt and loss, and make reparation
	Patient comes to be able to tolerate ambivalence in areas of conflict and to contain conflictual object relations within his sense of self

- *Interpretation conveying the inevitability of conflict:* Both the cognitive and affective components of insight and working through involve tolerating awareness of, and ultimately accepting, the inevitability of conflictual aspects of self experience.
- *The linking of current conflicts to the developmental past to facilitate working through:* Once conflictual object relations have been contained, explored, and to some degree worked through, understanding the developmental origins of unconscious fantasies and conflicts, as well as their relationship to presenting symptoms and personality traits, further diminishes anxiety, increases mastery, and introduces greater flexibility.

In Table 4–2 we provide an overview of the therapeutic process of DPHP. The table provides an outline of the therapist's central tasks during the course of treatment. The therapist's tasks appear in the lefthand column of the table, in the order in which they are implemented during the course of treatment, moving from the top to the bottom of the page. The righthand column of Table 4–2 describes anticipated developments in the therapeutic process as a result of the therapist's interventions. These developments are described in terms of changes in the internal experience and capacities of the patient.

SUGGESTED READINGS

Cooper A: Changes in psychoanalytic ideas: transference interpretation. J Am Psychoanal Assoc 35:77–98, 1987

Fosshage J: Toward reconceptualizing transference: theoretical and clinical considerations. Int J Psychoanal 75:265–280, 1994

Freud S: The dynamics of transference (1912), in The Standard Edition of the Complete Psychological Works of Sigmund Freud, Vol 12. Edited and translated by Strachey J. London, Hogarth Press, 1958, pp 99–108

Freud S: Observations on transference-love (1915), in The Standard Edition of the Complete Psychological Works of Sigmund Freud, Vol 12. Edited and translated by Strachey J. London, Hogarth Press, 1958, pp 159–171

Gabbard GO, Westen D: Rethinking therapeutic action. Int J Psychoanal 84:823–841, 2003

Gill M: Analysis of transference. J Am Psychoanal Assoc 27:263–288, 1979

Harris A: Transference, countertransference and the real relationship, in The American Psychiatric Publishing Textbook of Psychoanalysis. Washington, DC, American Psychiatric Publishing, 2005, pp 201–216

Høgland P, Amlo S, Marble A, et al: Analysis of the patient-therapist relationship in dynamic psychotherapy: an experimental study of transference interpretation. Am J Psychiatry 163:1739–1746, 2006

Joseph B: Transference: the total situation. Int J Psychoanal 66:447–454, 1985

Kernberg OF: An ego psychology-object relations theory approach to the transference, in Aggression in Personality Disorders and Perversions, 1992, pp 119–139

Loewald H: On the therapeutic action of psychoanalysis. Int J Psychoanal 41:16–33, 1960

Schafer R: The analytic attitude: an introduction, in The Analytic Attitude. New York, Basic Books, 1983, pp 3–13

Steiner J: The aim of psychoanalysis in theory and practice. Int J Psychoanal 77:1073–1083, 1996

Steiner J: Interpretive enactments and the analytic setting (with comments by Edgar Levenson). Int J Psychoanal 87:315–328, 2006

Westen D, Gabbard G: Developments in cognitive neuroscience, II: implications for theories of transference. J Am Psychoanal Assoc 50:99–134, 2002

THE STRATEGIES OF DPHP
AND THE TREATMENT SETTING

This chapter presents the strategies of dynamic psychotherapy for higher level personality pathology (DPHP) and describes the treatment frame. "Treatment strategies" refers to the long-range objectives of the treatment and the fundamental technical principles underlying the treatment as a whole. *Strategies* define the therapeutic approach the therapist employs to help the patient move toward progressive integration of conflictual object relations. The treatment strategies of DPHP are firmly embedded in the model of the mind and of unconscious conflict that we have presented. The strategies of the treatment are reflected in *tactics* that guide decision making regarding interventions in every treatment hour. *Techniques* are the consistent ways in which interventions are constructed and applied during the entire treatment. The strategies, tactics, and techniques of DPHP define a theory of psychotherapeutic technique.

The treatment setting of DPHP is designed to enable therapist and patient to implement the treatment strategies; the psychotherapeutic setting provides the context within which our theory of technique becomes a treatment. In DPHP, the psychotherapeutic setting creates a stable and predictable environment for the therapy while fostering an atmosphere of safety.

In the second half of this chapter, we discuss the treatment setting and the "treatment frame." The treatment frame defines the necessary conditions for the treatment and the respective roles of patient and therapist. The treatment frame contains the psychotherapeutic relationship, an essential vehicle for the treatment. We discuss the functions and specific features of the treatment frame and the psychotherapeutic relationship. We also introduce the therapeutic alliance, an aspect of the relationship between patient and therapist that plays a central role in all forms of psychotherapy.

OVERVIEW OF STRATEGIES

The overriding goal of DPHP is to introduce a greater degree of flexibility into those aspects of the patient's defensive operations that are responsible for symptoms and maladaptive personality traits. This is accomplished, first, by helping the patient to consciously tolerate awareness of repressed and dissociated object relations connected to presenting complaints, and, second, by helping the patient to assimilate these conflictual object relations into his dominant sense of self, so that they become part of his subjective experience.

The strategy that we employ in DPHP is to explore the object relations enacted in the treatment. We begin with defensively activated object relations and move toward the more threatening and affectively charged object relations being defended against. In this process, conflictual object relations underlying the patient's presenting complaints are brought to consciousness, and the conflicts embedded in conflictual representations of self and other can be explored, interpreted, and worked through.

Conflictual object relations tend to be activated and enacted in current interpersonal relationships. As a result, when listening to his patient, the DPHP therapist will typically be able to identify one or two relationship patterns that are salient in any given session, enacted in the patient's descriptions of his interactions with others and/or in the patient's interactions with the therapist. Having identified the object relations dominant in the session, the therapist will describe them and will help the patient explore the conflicts embedded in these object relations. As conflicts are enacted, explored, and interpreted, repeatedly over time, the object relations associated with these conflicts will be modified, becoming better integrated and less threatening, so that they can be assimilated into the patient's dominant self experience.

As the therapist explores the conflicts embedded in the patient's object relations, he keeps the treatment goals in mind. In DPHP, we focus on the relationship between the patient's conflicts and the treatment goals, addressing personality rigidity in localized areas of maladaptive functioning while leaving areas of relatively unimpaired functioning undisturbed.

TABLE 5–1. Strategies of dynamic psychotherapy for higher level
personality pathology (DPHP)

Strategy 1	Defining the dominant object relations
Strategy 2	Exploring and interpreting the conflicts and defenses embedded in the dominant object relations
Strategy 3	Narrowing the focus to the treatment goals
Strategy 4	Working through identified conflicts: integrating conflictual object relations into the patient's conscious self experience

---

When making interpretations, the therapist focuses on the relationship between the conflictual object relations being enacted and the patient's goals. The strategies used in DPHP (Table 5–1) can be conceptualized in terms of four sequential tasks, which we describe below.

STRATEGY 1: DEFINING THE DOMINANT OBJECT RELATIONS

The first strategy in DPHP is to define the dominant representations of self and other active in the session. While it can be tempting to think of mental representations as concrete entities, it is important to remember that they are not. Rather, mental representations and internal object relations are a person's customary way of organizing his experience of himself and of his internal and external reality. Internal object relations cannot be directly observed, and the nature of the representations of self and other active at any given moment can only be inferred from the ways in which they shape the patient's thoughts, feelings, and behaviors, and in particular his experience of and interactions with others. In DPHP, we make inferences about the patient's internal object world on the basis of his verbal and nonverbal communications. As we try to define the self and object representations currently dominant, we pay special attention to the patient's descriptions of interpersonal interactions, listening for the relationship patterns activated in the patient's interactions with others, including the patient's interactions with the therapist.

STEP 1: IDENTIFYING THE DOMINANT OBJECT RELATIONS

As he listens to and interacts with his patient, the DPHP therapist will construct hypotheses about the internal object relations currently being enacted. At this stage it can be helpful for the therapist to imagine, quite literally, an image of two people in interaction, each playing a particular

role. Typically the patient will be predominantly identified with one particular role in any given conflictual relationship pattern, although at times his
identification with both sides of a relationship pattern (or of all three, in the
case of triadic relationship patterns) may be quite close to consciousness.
This type of flexibility, though, is more commonly seen later in treatment
or after a particular conflict has been to some degree worked through.

In DPHP, we want our descriptions of the patient's mental representations to be as specific and as accurate as possible. In order to accurately identify the self and object representations currently active, the therapist will
need to have considerable information about the patient's current feelings,
wishes, and fears, along with his current experience and expectations of the
therapy and the therapist. The therapist gathers this information by listening closely to what the patient is saying, by observing the nonverbal interactions between the patient and the therapist, and by attending carefully to
his own private reactions to the patient in the session (Kernberg 1992). This
information will be integrated with the therapist's previous knowledge of the
patient, including his presenting problems and his developmental history.

When the therapist feels that a particular object relation is starting to
come into focus, he will ask for additional details about the person or interaction the patient is describing. If something remains unclear, the therapist
can share his uncertainty with the patient while asking the patient to help
resolve the therapist's lack of understanding. If the object relation coming
into focus is being enacted in the interaction with the therapist, the therapist
can explore the nature of the patient's experience of the interaction between
them. As a particular relationship pattern is coming into focus, it is often
helpful for the therapist to describe back to the patient some of the features
that apparently characterize the representations being enacted, to see if the
therapist has an accurate understanding of the patient's communications.

CLINICAL ILLUSTRATION OF IDENTIFYING
THE DOMINANT OBJECT RELATION

A 34-year-old professional woman, well loved by friends and colleagues, but
single while hoping for marriage and children, came to treatment complaining of dissatisfaction with her romantic life. The patient had, for the past
2 years, been infatuated with a male colleague, a man who frequently spent
time with her and flirted with her, but had no interest in her as a serious romantic partner. The patient knew the relationship was not good for her and
was most likely going nowhere, but she couldn't let it go. Friends had urged
her to give up on him, but she could not follow their good advice. Other
men had approached her, but she found them uninteresting.

At the urging of her friends, the patient began in treatment. She had
been in treatment for several months and had spent most of the current ses-

sion describing her date the previous evening with her colleague. She went on to say that even though she still longed to be with him, lately she found that she was not able to fully enjoy their time together. She was too aware of the fact that he did not give her his full attention or his full affection. She felt that although he had more to give, he would not give it to her.

The patient went on to acknowledge that she was beginning to experience this man as actively withholding from her, and at times she found herself wondering if this was something he was doing on purpose. As he listened, the therapist noted a tone of frustration in the patient's voice. In his mind, the therapist identified the patient's experience with her colleague, as she had just described it, as the dominant object relation activated in the session.

STEP 2: NAMING THE ACTORS

Once the therapist has an opinion about the object relation being enacted, he will share his impression with the patient. It is generally optimal to do this at a point when the patient has alluded to a particular object relation or theme repeatedly in a session, or when variations of a particular object relation have emerged in more than one form. Alternatively, the therapist should intervene when he notices that the dominant relationship pattern in the patient's verbal communications is simultaneously being enacted in the patient's interactions with the therapist.

In deciding when to intervene, the therapist pays attention to the patient's affective state. It is most effective to describe a particular object relation at a time when the patient is feeling emotionally involved in some aspect of the interaction the therapist is naming. The major exception to this rule is that it is generally not optimal to "name the actors" at a moment of peak affective intensity. If an object relation comes into clear focus at a time when the patient's affects are extremely intense, we recommend that the therapist wait until the patient is calmer before trying to shed light on the underlying self and object representations that are being enacted. This is because extremely intense affects often compromise the capacity for self-reflection. Once the patient no longer feels "swept away," he will be more open to hearing a description of the object relations underlying the intensity of his affective experience.

When naming the "actors" in a particular relationship pattern, the therapist's stance is nonjudgmental. His aim is to be accepting of all aspects of the patient's experience, and to convey neither criticism nor approval. The therapist maintains this stance even when a particular role is objectively objectionable or desirable. For example, when approaching the relationship pattern of the frustrated patient-self and the withholding man-object, the therapist will describe the attributes of the two actors without implying that the boyfriend is bad or that the patient is either to be admired or pitied. When naming the actors, the therapist is also nonauthoritarian. The therapist is presenting a hypothesis, to be tested and refined on the basis of the patient's response, not a truth that is to be necessarily accepted by the patient. In this spirit, it is often helpful for the therapist to share with the patient the thinking that led him to this hypothesis (Busch 1996).

When describing an object relation to a patient, the therapist should look for and include in his description particular details that specifically characterize the actors and what is taking place between them. Using the patient's own language can be very helpful in this regard and can bring representations of self and other to life in an especially vivid and emotionally rich fashion. To illustrate this approach, let's return to the session described above, in which our patient describes having difficulty enjoying her time with her man friend.

CLINICAL ILLUSTRATION OF NAMING THE ACTORS

After listening to the patient, clarifying her experience of the evening before, and exploring her reflections on the evening, the therapist makes an attempt to describe the actors. For example, the therapist might say to the patient, "It seems that you are having a particular experience of your interactions with this man. Even if this is not his actual intention, it sounds like you are starting to feel that he is purposefully withholding from you, almost as if he *wants* to frustrate you. Is this an accurate description of how you feel?"

If this impression proves correct, the therapist might then proceed to name the actors. The therapist might suggest to the patient, "It is as if you have in your mind a particular image of two people in interaction. One person is waiting for love and attention from someone important to them. The other person is not fully available, and, further, is secretly aware of withholding from and frustrating the first person."

STEP 3: ATTENDING TO THE PATIENT'S REACTION

After offering a particular hypothesis about the object relation currently active, the therapist will attend carefully to the patient's reaction to his comments. In listening to a patient's response, the therapist will care less about the patient's manifest agreement or disagreement and more about the patient's subsequent associations and behavior. The therapist can hear the material that follows as expressions of the patient's reactions to the therapist's intervention. If, during this process, the therapist comes to realize that his inference was off the mark, he should feel free to acknowledge this and to provide a revised impression as it emerges.

A correct characterization of the predominant object relation may lead to several possible developments. Sometimes the patient will acknowledge, with emotional conviction, recognition of what the therapist is describing. The patient may spontaneously describe other interactions showing a similar pattern, or he may respond by associating to material or memories related to the object relation the therapist has described. This process may add new dimensions to the object relation in question. For example, our patient with relationship problems might spontaneously associate to a childhood pattern of frustrating interactions with a sibling. Alternatively, an article in the paper about mothers who neglect their children may come to mind, suggesting that the frustrating relationship with her boyfriend is connected to an image of a parent and child in interaction.

Sometimes a patient will respond to a correct characterization of the predominant object relation by enacting that relationship with the therapist; the patient we have been describing might respond by complaining how frustrating it is to be in this kind of therapy, where she gets so little feedback or direction from the therapist.

At other times, the patient may respond by associating to the described object relation but reversing the roles. In this situation, our patient might start talking about an anecdote in which someone accused her of using withholding or frustrating behavior, or she might associate to a shameful childhood memory of teasing a household pet. Or the patient may reverse the roles in relation to the therapist—for example, by ignoring the therapist's intervention or in a teasing way communicating that she has something on her mind that she is not sharing. Sometimes a correct characterization will lead to the sudden activation of a different object relation that reflects other aspects of the current conflict—for example, images of self and other that are closer to the impulses being defended against or represent the anxiety motivating defense.

STRATEGY 2: OBSERVING AND INTERPRETING THE CONFLICTS EMBEDDED IN THE DOMINANT OBJECT RELATIONS

We have noted that the first strategy of DPHP is to identify, describe, and explore the object relations that are dominant in the patient's verbal and nonverbal communications. The therapist's next strategy is to develop a hypothesis about the psychological conflicts embedded in the object relations that have been described and explored, and to share this hypothesis with the patient in the form of an interpretation.

In higher level personality pathology, the internal object relations associated with conflictual motivations, be they wishes, needs, or fears, are predominantly out of the patient's awareness, and they tend to remain so. The patient's defensive organization, which involves enacting and consciously experiencing a particular constellation of object relations in a particular configuration, is also quite stable. As a result, in the normal course of events the patient will enact defensive internal object relations while remaining largely, if not entirely, unaware of conflictual motivations and associated object relations until they are activated and explored in treatment.

As we have described, there are a number of ways that internal object relations can be used to defend against psychological conflict. First, enactment of relatively acceptable object relations can be used defensively, to support repression of underlying conflictual motivations. Second, enactment of any internal object relation in which a threatening need, wish, or fear is attributed to an object representation while dissociated from the self serves as a compromise formation in relation to the threatening impulse. Third, enactment of conflictual object relations that are split off or dissociated from dominant self experience allows for expression of conflictual motivations while sidestepping the anxieties associated with the underlying conflict.

Returning to our example of the patient with relationship problems, close to consciousness and repeatedly enacted is an object relation of a dependent and loving self and an unavailable and withholding object, associated with feelings of frustration. Enactment of this relationship pattern supports repression of underlying object relations that are more threatening and more closely tied to the expression of underlying oedipally colored, erotic desires. Enactment of the relationship pattern of a dependent self and a withholding object additionally serves as a compromise formation in relation to the patient's own impulses to frustrate and withhold from someone more vulnerable. Finally, enacting the relationship pattern of a withholding self and a dependent object, while dissociating these object relations from dominant self experience and denying their significance, allows the patient to express motivations to frustrate and withhold, while avoiding conflict.

STEP 1: IDENTIFYING AND EXPLORING DEFENSIVE INTERNAL OBJECT RELATIONS

The first step in exploring a conflict is to identify, describe, and explore the object relation dominant in the session—beginning with naming the actors, as described above. In our example, the therapist would help the patient appreciate that she repeatedly enacts a situation in which she feels like a dependent, needy, and loving child in relation to an unavailable and withholding object, and that this leads to chronic feelings of frustration. As this defensive enactment is identified and explored, in the patient's interpersonal relationships and perhaps in relation to the therapist as well, it can be identified as serving defensive functions. By this, we mean that the patient will come to appreciate that she repeatedly *constructs* this situation, either in fantasy or in reality.

Identification and exploration of defensive object relations as they are enacted in the patient's interpersonal life and in the transference will slowly lead to changes in the patient's attitude toward these defensive enactments. First, the patient will become aware of aspects of his behavior that he had previously not paid attention to, and second, he will become aware that *he is an active participant in creating the interpersonal situations he repeatedly "finds" himself in.* Returning to our patient, she will come to appreciate that being dependent and frustrated is not something that entirely happens "to" the patient, but rather is an interpersonal experience that she actively and repeatedly participates in creating.

Once a patient appreciates that he is actively, albeit unknowingly and automatically, putting himself in particular situations, it generally leads to curiosity on the part of the patient as to what would be motivating his behavior. As the patient comes to appreciate the ways in which he repeatedly does things that leave him feeling a certain way, the therapist will raise the question of why the patient would be choosing to do the things he is. Returning to our clinical example, the therapist would help the patient to consider the question of why she would be choosing, out of her awareness and beyond her control, to put herself in such a chronically frustrating position.

As a result of identifying and exploring a particular cluster of defensive object relations, the patient will become curious about why she behaves as she does, and she will come to appreciate that her behavior is driven by motivations that are out of her awareness. At the same time, enactment of the defensive relationship pattern will become not only more visible to the patient (i.e., it will become "ego dystonic"), but also less effective in protecting the patient from awareness of the anxieties and motivations defended against.

STEP 2: IDENTIFYING AND EXPLORING CONFLICTUAL OBJECT RELATIONS

As the patient's defenses become more visible to the patient and less rigid, they will become less effective at keeping underlying conflicts entirely out of the patient's conscious awareness. In this setting, relationship patterns that are derivatives of the anxieties and conflicts being defended against will begin to appear in the patient's verbal and nonverbal communications. This opens the door to the identification and exploration of previously repressed or dissociated object relations. Typically, the object relations that have been defended against will be more closely or directly tied to expression of conflictual motivations than are the defensively activated object relations. As the clusters of object relations associated with a particular need, fear, or wish are identified and described, the therapist can begin to form hypotheses about the nature of the patient's core conflicts, sharing them with the patient in the form of preliminary interpretations.

CLINICAL ILLUSTRATION OF IDENTIFYING AND EXPLORING CONFLICTUAL OBJECT RELATIONS

After spending several sessions exploring her tendency to put herself in the position of feeling dependent and frustrated, the patient described above told her therapist that she had been asked out by a new man, a long-standing admirer. The therapist noted that as the patient spoke of the man and his invitation, her tone was casually dismissive. In the patient's attitude toward her admirer, the therapist identified an enactment of the relationship pattern that they had been exploring in the treatment, but with the roles reversed.

The therapist pointed this out to the patient and described the relationship pattern in which, faced with someone whom she perceives as admiring of her, the patient experienced the person as "needy" and was stimulated to behave in a withholding and ultimately frustrating fashion. In response, the patient acknowledged a long-standing pattern in which, without thinking about it, she was quietly and politely inaccessible to her admirers, leaving them feeling dismissed and frustrated by her lack of interest. This was something about herself that the patient had been vaguely aware of but had never really thought about until now; it seemed to have little to do with her overall view of herself. In the treatment, therapist and patient explored this aspect of the patient's interactions with men. They linked the feelings of self-criticism and low mood that the patient often experienced in response to receiving attention from men to her discomfort with her own impulses to be frustrating and withholding toward someone she perceived as needy.

Typically, as a patient works through the more accessible aspects of a particular constellation of conflicts, other, more deeply repressed aspects of the conflict will be activated and will become detectable in the material. For example, first, the patient we have been describing began to work through her conflictual motivations to frustrate people whom she saw as less powerful than herself. As she became more tolerant of these motives, she began to be aware of anxiety and guilt associated with allowing herself to feel more sexually desirable. Ultimately, her guilt and anxiety proved to be linked to unacceptable wishes to use her sexual attractiveness to feel powerful.

In this setting, the therapist was able to point out that by experiencing herself as either frustrated or frustrating, the patient had avoided whatever anxiety she might feel if she were to experience herself as sexually desirable to a desirable man. Exploration of this anxiety opened the door to uncovering unacceptable, unconscious wishes and fantasies of receiving sexual attention and admiration from a powerful man while excluding and triumphing over a less desirable woman. Here, the impulsive internal object relation involved a triangular situation of a sexually powerful self who is pleasurably getting attention from a powerful man while excluding and humiliating a less desirable woman. When she came to treatment, the patient had been defending against enactment of this highly conflictual object relation, closely tied to sexual, competitive, and sadistic oedipal impulses, by feeling like a loving, frustrated child.

The internal object relations associated with expression of unconscious wishes, needs, and fears tend to be highly affectively charged, and the representations involved can be extremely threatening to the patient. These internal object relations and associated fantasies will be largely, if not entirely, outside the patient's awareness until they are uncovered and explored in the treatment. It is the job of the DPHP therapist to describe and explore these threatening object relations and affect states from a position of technical neutrality, while acknowledging the anxiety, fear, guilt, loss, or shame associated with their expression. This stance on the part of the therapist will help the patient tolerate and contain painful awareness of emotionally threatening aspects of his inner life that previously had been rejected from conscious self experience.

STRATEGY 3: NARROWING THE FOCUS TO THE TREATMENT GOALS

As we have discussed, DPHP is a treatment organized around specific treatment goals, agreed upon as part of the consultative process. In DPHP, we have modified standard psychoanalytic technique by narrowing the treatment goals of DPHP relative to psychoanalysis. This makes it possible to conduct successful treatments that are shorter and less intensive than psychoanalysis, but nonetheless effective in a specific area of functioning. Where a psychoanalytic treatment will explore comprehensively the patient's inner life and conflicts, DPHP will explore the patient's core conflicts, with an emphasis on their relationship to the patient's presenting problems and the treatment goals. Where a psychoanalytic treatment is oriented toward integration of conflictual object relations responsible for personality rigidity at large, DPHP is oriented toward integration of conflictual object relations in circumscribed areas of functioning. As a result, as the therapist explores the dominant object relations, he always has an eye on the patient's current reality, presenting complaints, and treatment goals.

EMPHASIZING THE RELATIONSHIP BETWEEN CORE CONFLICTS AND THE TREATMENT GOALS

Every patient has core or dominant conflicts that will be enacted in the treatment. These conflicts affect the patient in many areas of functioning—

in some areas very powerfully, in others much more subtly. In DPHP, as a particular conflict comes into focus, the therapist will be thinking to himself, "How might these relationship patterns relate to the patient's presenting problems and treatment goals?" When exploring a conflict with the patient, the therapist will emphasize the relationship between that conflict and the patient's personality rigidity in the circumscribed areas designated in the treatment goals. This process offers the opportunity to develop a deeper understanding of the problems that brought the patient to treatment and to work through anxieties underlying presenting complaints, by focusing therapeutically on areas of functioning of particular concern to the patient—while leaving areas of relatively intact functioning unexplored.

Returning to our patient in the frustrating relationship: in order to focus on the treatment goals, the therapist will emphasize the relationship between the object relations activated in the treatment and the patient's difficulty in achieving intimacy with a suitable partner. These same object relations could easily and accurately be linked to the patient's competitive conflicts about success in the workplace, as well as her tendency to hold herself to excessively high standards. However, in exploring the dominant object relations and the conflicts embedded in them, the therapist consistently emphasized the patient's conflicts involving intimacy while leaving related conflicts involving professional success and self-criticism relatively unattended.

The strategy of emphasizing the link between the patient's core conflicts and the treatment goals may be the therapeutic task in DPHP that most powerfully requires what is often referred to as "clinical judgment." However, a core premise of our overall approach is that it is possible to operationalize the principles underlying clinical judgment. In this particular context, the task requiring "clinical judgment" is to bring proper timing and emphasis to the tactic of focusing on circumscribed areas of personality rigidity by interpreting the relationship between the conflicts dominant in the treatment and the treatment goals.

What are the technical implications of the therapist's "focusing" his interpretations? At what point in the process of analyzing a particular conflict should the therapist introduce the treatment goals? How powerfully, at any given point, should the therapist emphasize the link between the dominant conflict and the treatment goals? These are questions that we will explore in depth in Chapter 8, "The Tactics of DPHP." In general, it is the process of "working through" that presents opportunity for focusing on the relationship between core conflicts and the treatment goals.

STRATEGY 4: WORKING THROUGH OF IDENTIFIED CONFLICTS—INTEGRATING CONFLICTUAL OBJECT RELATIONS INTO THE PATIENT'S CONSCIOUS SELF EXPERIENCE

The final strategy of DPHP is to promote the assimilation of conflictual object relations into the patient's subjective experience and his dominant sense of self. For the patient whom we have been discussing, this would entail first coming to tolerate awareness of her wishes to frustrate and withhold, accepting these wishes as her own and integrating them into a sense of herself as a complex person with complex motivations and fears. Second, in a similar fashion, the patient would become aware of and come to tolerate her wishes to triumph sexually. As she is able to tolerate awareness of wishes to frustrate, the patient will no longer need to defensively put herself in the position of being frustrated. As she becomes aware of her wishes to triumph sexually and is able to better integrate these object relations and assimilate them into her dominant self experience, she will be free to enjoy admiration, love, and sexual attention from a man whom she admires. Her wishes for oedipal triumph, now embedded in her overall sense of herself as a loving and decent person, can be expressed and enjoyed as part of her erotic life.

WORKING THROUGH AND THE PROCESS OF CHANGE

In DPHP, integration of internal object relations does not result simply from interpretation, or even from insight. Rather, integration is the fruit of repeated enactment, containment, exploration, and interpretation, in an emotionally meaningful fashion, of the defenses and anxieties associated with the expression of conflictual object relations. This is the process of *working through*. In this process, it is necessary to enact and explore the object relations that represent the defenses and anxieties associated with expression of a particular conflictual motivation from a variety of perspectives and in a variety of contexts. Typically this process takes place over the course of months and is then followed by intermittent reactivation and further working through of the same cluster of internal object relations throughout the course of treatment.

In DPHP, we expect that a particular conflict will be repeatedly activated and enacted in the treatment, at times seemingly put to rest only to reappear down the road in another context. On each such occasion, the internal object relations representing the defensive side of a conflict will be explored and interpreted, and the patient will come to tolerate awareness of the underlying object relations defended against. Over time, as object relations associated with core conflicts become familiar to patient and therapist and are increasingly well

tolerated by the patient, it becomes possible to identify and interpret a particular conflict with increasing ease and in a more condensed period of time. As
treatment progresses, a conflict initially analyzed over the course of weeks, or
even months, can be explored and interpreted in the course of a single session.

Tolerating awareness of conflictual internal object relations paves the
way for taking responsibility for conflictual aspects of the self and mourning
losses associated with acknowledging psychological conflicts. The outcome
is that the individual consciously tolerates awareness of conflictual motivations and associated anxieties and is able to cope with them in a flexible fashion that does not rely on repression, dissociation, projection, or denial. It is
the process of repeated enactment and working through of a conflict over
the course of the entire treatment—accompanied by a progressive capacity
to tolerate, contain, and take responsibility for conflictual object relations
and associated anxieties and fantasies—that leads to structural change.

In the process of working through, the therapist emphasizes the relationship between core conflicts and the treatment goals, placing less emphasis on the ways in which core conflicts affect other areas of functioning.
In addition, we expect that, at some point in the process of working
through, aspects of core conflicts will be worked through in the transference. Even with patients who are highly resistant to transference interpretations, the process of working through almost always provides opportunity
to make a meaningful link between the patient's dominant conflicts and his
experience of and/or behavior with the therapist.

THE TREATMENT SETTING AND THE TREATMENT FRAME

The treatment setting of DPHP is designed to enable therapist and patient
to implement the treatment strategies. The psychotherapeutic setting provides a stable and reliable environment for the treatment while fostering an
atmosphere of safety. The *treatment frame* defines the necessary conditions
for the treatment. The frame establishes the respective tasks of patient and
therapist in the treatment as well as the steady and predictable structure of
the psychotherapeutic setting. The treatment frame is mutually agreed
upon by patient and therapist before treatment begins. The agreement between therapist and patient that establishes the treatment frame is often referred to as the *treatment contract* (Clarkin et al. 2006; Etchegoyen 1991).

As we will describe in Chapter 9 ("Patient Assessment and Differential
Treatment Planning"), before beginning treatment the therapist will provide
a complete consultation. This process entails the therapist's 1) doing a diagnostic evaluation, 2) sharing his diagnostic impression with the patient, 3) clarifying the patient's treatment goals and 4) discussing treatment options. In the

process of discussing treatment options, the therapist will have provided a description of DPHP. (We provide detailed description of the consultative process in Chapter 9.) If at the end of the consultation the patient decides that he wants to begin in DPHP, the therapist introduces the treatment frame, including concrete arrangements and the respective roles of patient and therapist.

Establishing the treatment frame is an important part of the process of initiating treatment. Discussion of the frame enables the patient to begin the treatment with a clear expectation of what the treatment entails and a clear understanding of the respective roles of patient and therapist in a process designed to enable the patient to attain his specified treatment goals. The treatment frame and the treatment contract serve a variety of functions in the opening phase and throughout the course of treatment, and maintaining the treatment frame is an essential responsibility of both patient and therapist in DPHP. When there is a disruption of the treatment frame, analyzing the meaning of the disruption becomes a priority theme in the session.

THE FUNCTIONS OF THE TREATMENT FRAME IN DPHP

Before beginning treatment, the therapist will discuss the treatment contract with the patient. Introducing the treatment frame during the consultation will often bring to light whatever anxieties the patient has in relation to beginning treatment. These anxieties will typically be activated in the transference and/ or will touch on the patient's core conflicts. If a patient expresses interest in DPHP but then is unable or unwilling to agree to the treatment contract, exploration of the patient's concerns about the treatment frame can shed light on the anxieties underlying his presenting complaints. In this setting, the therapist's capacity to tactfully, empathically, and neutrally clarify and explore the fears activated around agreeing to the treatment frame will help to solidify the treatment alliance, as well as help the patient to contain his anxiety. Exploration of a patient's reluctance to agree to the treatment frame also will enable the therapist to distinguish between the patient who is ambivalent about treatment and needs help working though his anxieties about beginning DPHP and the patient who is not currently suited for DPHP, given his current level of motivation for treatment or his current life circumstances.

CLINICAL ILLUSTRATION OF
ESTABLISHING THE TREATMENT FRAME

A 55-year-old woman, recently divorced after a long and unhappy marriage, presented with "problems with relationships." The patient was interested in DPHP until she understood that the treatment could not be done on a once-a-week basis. Her initial reaction was to feel strongly that the consultant's recommendation of a twice-weekly treatment was "outrageous" and would be "impossible" given the demands of her work schedule.

Rather than simply taking the patient's reaction at face value, the therapist tried to help her clarify the thoughts and feelings behind her very powerful reaction to the suggestion of a twice-a-week schedule. As the therapist encouraged the patient to reflect on her difficulty with considering a twice-weekly treatment and helped her to explore what she imagined would happen in such a treatment, it emerged that the patient assumed that the therapist would insist on the patient's coming at times convenient for the therapist while paying no attention to demands of the patient's schedule. Therapist and patient were able to clarify the patient's conscious but unexamined expectation that the only way she could obtain help with her problems was to submit entirely to a powerful figure, in this case the therapist, completely abdicating her own needs. The therapist was able quite easily to link this expectation to a relationship pattern that had been played out chronically in the patient's marriage.

The process of establishing and clearly explaining the treatment frame before beginning treatment can facilitate the formation of a treatment alliance (the treatment alliance is discussed later in this chapter). Description of the frame and explanation of the rationale for aspects of the frame that may not be self-evident also helps to demystify the psychotherapeutic process, enlisting the patient's full and active participation. In essence, patients can only do what they are asked to do, and they do it more effectively if they understand the rationale for what they are doing. Carefully reviewing and explaining the rationale for the treatment contract can facilitate the patient's moving efficiently through the tasks of the opening phase of treatment (described in Chapter 10, "The Phases of Treatment").

Once treatment begins, the treatment frame serves the important function of providing a setting that is reliable and consistent in its structure and predictable with regard to the roles played by therapist and patient. This consistency and predictability is part of the atmosphere of safety provided by the psychotherapeutic setting. It is only when the setting is objectively "safe" that it becomes reasonable for a patient to open himself up to the therapist and attempt to examine his inner experience and anxieties in the therapist's presence.

Throughout the course of treatment, the treatment frame provides a steady setting and set of expectations for conducting the treatment that will highlight even subtle deviations from "business as usual" and will make it possible to view deviations from the frame as having meaning. This is to say that in DPHP the patient's relationship to the treatment frame and the treatment contract is twofold. On the one hand, the patient consciously accepts the treatment contract and the tasks of patient and therapist in the psychotherapeutic relationship as the therapist has explained them. On the other hand, the patient will invariably come upon difficulty maintaining the treatment frame. Our general approach is that the more clearly the patient understands the conditions of the treatment as well as the rationale for structuring the treatment in the way that we do, the easier it is to explore the meanings of the patient's wishes to modify the frame once treatment begins. Similarly, a clearly defined frame will help the therapist to identify subtle countertranferences, expressed as wishes to somehow deviate from or modify the treatment frame.

Maintaining the integrity of the treatment frame is an essential component of any form of treatment. In DPHP, if the integrity of the frame is violated either intentionally or unwittingly, by patient or therapist, exploring the meanings of the deviation becomes a priority theme in the session.

SPECIFIC FEATURES OF THE TREATMENT FRAME IN DPHP

The treatment frame defines the concrete arrangements of the treatment and the respective tasks of patient and therapist in the psychotherapeutic relationship. Concrete arrangements to be discussed before beginning treatment include the frequency and duration of sessions, arrangements for handling scheduling and payment, and expectations about contact, either on the phone or face to face, between patient and therapist outside of regularly scheduled appointments.

In DPHP, sessions are twice weekly, usually last 45 or 50 minutes and begin and end on time. Patient and therapist sit across from one another, face to face, in comfortable chairs. Appointments are typically scheduled for the same day and time each week, but this can be modified if need be to accommodate the schedules of patient and therapist. What is important is that standard procedures for scheduling appointments are established at the beginning of treatment and that appointments are scheduled ahead of time and not on an as-needed or last-minute basis, except in extraordinary circumstances. Phone calls and contact between sessions is typically limited to schedule changes and emergencies; patients are encouraged to discuss even urgent matters in session, rather than calling between sessions.

Every therapist should have standard arrangements for handling logistics in the treatment that he can clearly explain to the patient before treatment begins. Procedures should include how appointments are scheduled and rescheduled, how the patient will be billed, and the expectations with regard to payment, how to contact the therapist, and what the patient can expect with regard to the therapist's procedures for returning phone calls. The rationale for establishing standard procedures is to quickly bring it to the therapist's attention when he is feeling tempted to modify his usual approach. This recognition on the part of the therapist then opens the door to the use of countertransference as a source of information about what is going on in the current clinical situation.

In addition to specifying the concrete arrangements of the treatment, the treatment contract also defines the respective tasks of the therapist and patient in the therapy. In DPHP it is the patient's task to attend sessions regularly, to handle logistics in the fashion outlined by the therapist at the beginning of treatment, and to speak as openly and freely as possible about what is going through his mind during his therapy sessions. It is the therapist's task to adhere to the logistical arrangements agreed upon at the beginning of treatment and, once treatment begins, to listen attentively to the patient and to intervene when there is opportunity to deepen the patient's understanding of his inner situation.

INTRODUCING THE TREATMENT FRAME AND THE RESPECTIVE ROLES OF PATIENT AND THERAPIST

When introducing the treatment frame, the therapist can begin by explaining how logistics are handled and the responsibilities of patient and therapist in relation to how appointments are scheduled and rescheduled, how the patient will be billed and expectations with regard to payment, how to contact the therapist, and how the therapist returns phone calls. Once these concrete aspects of the frame are introduced, the therapist will move on to describe the respective roles of patient and therapist in the therapy sessions. We recommend that when introducing the treatment frame the therapist invite questions about and offer explanation for the rationale of structuring the treatment in the manner he is suggesting. This approach fosters a collaborative atmosphere as the treatment begins.

Each therapist should develop his own way of introducing the respective roles of patient and therapist in the treatment. As an example, the therapist might say something like:

> "Let me explain the role that each of us will play in your therapy sessions. Your role is to attend sessions regularly and to speak as openly and freely as you can when you are here, without relying on a prepared agenda, paying special attention to the difficulties that brought you to treatment. I am asking you quite literally to try to say whatever goes through your mind and also to share with me whatever difficulty you may have doing so. I am suggesting that we work in this way because it is the best way I know of to learn about the thoughts and feelings that, out of your awareness, are underlying your difficulties.
>
> "At times, you may find that the thoughts you have in session seem trivial or embarrassing, but I would encourage you to share them even so. Similarly,

if you have thoughts or questions about me, I would encourage you to share them as well, even when they may not be the kind of thing one would share in an ordinary social relationship. Things you find yourself thinking about as you are coming to or leaving your sessions may also be helpful to explore, as can be dreams, daydreams, and fantasies that you have between sessions.

"What I am asking you to do is not so easy, and you will find at times that you are not comfortable being open or do not know what to say. This shouldn't be surprising; unless you've been in therapy before, you probably have never tried to communicate with someone in this way and for the express purpose of learning more about yourself. In fact, understanding whatever is interfering with your thinking and communicating freely and openly is an important part of the therapy and helps us to better understand how your mind works.

"When you find you have difficulty, I will do what I can to help you understand what is getting in the way. Otherwise, my job is to listen attentively and to share my thoughts when I feel I have something to add that will help to deepen our understanding of the patterns of thinking, behavior, and fantasies that underlie your difficulties. You will find that there will be times when I talk a fair amount, and other times when I will be relatively silent. You will also find that I may not always answer your questions. This is not to be rude or to discourage your curiosity, but rather to focus on what are the thoughts and feelings behind the question. Finally, I want to stress that everything you tell me here is confidential. What questions do you have about what I have said?"

THE PSYCHOTHERAPEUTIC RELATIONSHIP

Within the reliable structure of the treatment setting, therapist and patient establish a special relationship, or object relation, which we refer to as the *psychotherapeutic relationship*. The psychotherapeutic relationship is a unique and highly specialized relationship unlike any other. In the psychotherapeutic relationship, it is the patient's role to communicate his inner needs as openly and fully as possible, while the therapist refrains from doing so. It is the role of the therapist to use his expertise to broaden and deepen the patient's self-awareness, while maintaining an attitude of respect for the patient's autonomy and concern for his well-being. The psychotherapeutic relationship is established by the therapist as part of the treatment contract and is an essential feature of the frame of DPHP.

THE FUNCTIONS OF THE PSYCHOTHERAPEUTIC RELATIONSHIP IN DPHP

The psychotherapeutic relationship is the necessary context within which the treatment described in this handbook can be provided. Like the logistical aspects of the treatment setting, the psychotherapeutic relationship can be seen as serving a dual function. First, it provides the patient with the experience of being in a relationship that is highly consistent, predictable, nonjudgmental, and focused almost exclusively on the needs of the patient. These aspects of the psychotherapeutic setting, along with the predictable and consistent nature of the structure of the treatment, contribute to the "background of safety" (Sandler 1959, 2003) that enables the patient to gradually open himself up to the therapist and facilitates exploration of aspects of the patient's inner experience that he has been previously unable to attend to.

In addition to providing a consistent and reliable setting for the treatment, the psychotherapeutic relationship also provides the "objective" relationship that will inevitably be distorted by the patient's transference and defensive operations. The treatment contract establishes an objective or realistic interpersonal relationship between a patient who needs and wants help and a therapist he trusts to have the knowledge and experience to be helpful (Kernberg 2004b; Loewald 1960). As the treatment proceeds, the unfolding of the patient's internal object relations will lead to distortions of this experience of the relationship between patient and therapist, and these distortions will typically be enacted in relation to the therapist. This is to say that once the patient consciously accepts the psychotherapeutic relationship as a condition for treatment, he begins to subtly distort that relationship on the basis of his transferences and his defensive operations. As these distortions of the psychotherapeutic relationship become visible in the treatment, they become a focus of exploration.

In sum, the psychotherapeutic relationship, in conjunction with the reliable features of the treatment setting, functions to provide both a "safe" setting within which the patient's internal object relations can unfold and an objective relationship that will be distorted as a result of the unfolding of the patient's object relations. As these distortions are identified, they are implicitly viewed against the background of the relationship between patient and therapist as it was initially defined in the treatment contract. In this way, the realistic relationship between patient and therapist established at the beginning of treatment serves as a reference point for both patient and therapist throughout the course of treatment.

SPECIFIC FEATURES OF THE PSYCHOTHERAPEUTIC RELATIONSHIP IN DPHP

The psychotherapeutic relationship is defined by the respective tasks of patient and therapist in the treatment. The patient's role is to communicate his thoughts and feelings as they emerge in the session, saying whatever comes to mind without censoring or preparing an agenda. He is invited to speak in an unstructured way, as freely and openly as possible. Thus even though the therapy has defined goals, in any given DPHP session we ask the patient to put aside any specific agenda and allow his mind to wander freely. The therapist can explain that thinking and communicating in the way he is inviting the patient to do is different from ordinary social discourse and may feel strange at first. There will be times when the patient may find it difficult to communicate openly and freely, and at these times the therapist will do what he can to help.

The therapist's role is to listen attentively and to contribute what he can to increase the patient's understanding of himself, and especially of the unconscious processes that underlie his presenting complaints. The therapist may add that in DPHP it is not part of the therapist's role to provide advice or encouragement or to talk about himself, as one would in an ordinary social relationship. The therapist can explain that by abstaining from assuming an openly supportive stance, he is enhancing his capacity to help the patient better understand himself and his problems.

DEVIATIONS FROM THE TREATMENT FRAME

On the one hand, the patient in DPHP consciously accepts the treatment contract and the tasks of patient and therapist as the therapist has explained them. On the other hand, the patient will invariably come upon difficulty in fully maintaining the treatment contract. In particular, patients find it difficult to adhere to the designated roles assigned to patient and therapist in the treatment contract. In addition, even though patients with higher level personality pathology are generally reliable about scheduling appointments, attending sessions, and paying bills, in DPHP they will not always adhere to the arrangements as agreed upon in the treatment contract. In fact, we expect that at some point in treatment, most patients will in some way deviate from the agreed-upon frame.

THE FUNCTIONS OF DEVIATIONS FROM THE TREATMENT FRAME IN DPHP

As we have discussed, it is important that the DPHP therapist clearly describe the treatment frame to the patient before beginning the therapy. The emphasis we place on clear and specific explication of the treatment frame should not be taken to imply that it is necessary to rigidly adhere to a particular treatment frame in DPHP, or that we are interested in controlling the patient's behavior per se. Rather, the DPHP therapist makes the frame explicit in order to create a setting in which deviations from the frame can be viewed as having meaning. In DPHP, deviations from the treatment frame bring the patient's conflictual self and object representations into the treatment, in the form of behavior. A clearly defined treatment frame serves the purpose of highlighting even subtle deviations on the part of the patient or the therapist. Deviations from the frame are often the first sign of transference and countertransference themes that are emerging in treatment.

SPECIFIC FEATURES OF DEVIATIONS FROM THE TREATMENT FRAME IN DPHP

Deviations from the treatment frame come in many forms. The examples we provide below illustrate deviations on the part of patient and the therapist from the agreed-upon arrangements for the treatment. More subtle and universal resistances to maintaining the respective roles of patient and therapist will ebb and flow throughout the course of every DPHP treatment. We refer here, for example, to difficulties communicating openly with the therapist (discussed in Chapter 10 in relation to the opening phase of treatment) and to invitations to the therapist to deviate from his usual role to be, for example, more directive or more supportive (discussed in relation to technical neutrality in Chapter 7, "The Techniques of DPHP, Part II—Intervening").

Deviations in relation to arrangements of the treatment as they define the treatment frame come in a variety of forms. Commonly encountered deviations include frequent cancellations (effectively decreasing the frequency of sessions), chronic lateness (effectively decreasing the duration of sessions), frequent requests for schedule changes, frequent phone calls, and delay of payment. It is only natural that a patient will occasionally be late or cancel sessions or delay payment. However, if these behaviors are recurrent or frequent, they are likely to be expressions of object relations being activated in the transference, and if this is the case the deviation from the frame should become a focus of exploration. Lying, attempting to initiate social contact or physical contact with the therapist, coming to sessions high or drunk, and invading the therapist's privacy are deviations from the treatment frame more commonly encountered in patients with severe personality disorders but are, rarely, also seen with patients with higher level personality pathology.

CLINICAL ILLUSTRATIONS OF DEVIATION FROM THE TREATMENT FRAME

After being in therapy for 6 months, a female patient began to come a few minutes late to her sessions, rationalizing that demands at work were making it difficult for her to get there on time. When her female therapist commented on the patient's behavior and began to explore its meaning, the patient stopped coming late. As soon as she resumed coming on time, the patient found herself waiting for the therapist in her waiting room. Sitting there, the patient became aware of powerful longings to see her therapist and to be physically close to her, feelings that she had been able to keep at bay by coming late. At the same time, the patient became aware of fears that the therapist would find the patient's feelings disagreeable and that if the therapist knew how the patient felt, she would be tempted to reject her.

In this situation, the relationship with the therapist had activated an object relation of a needful, dependent child and an unresponsive, rejecting parent, associated with feelings of shame. By coming late, the patient was defending against awareness of this object relation. When the therapist explored with the patient her deviation from the treatment frame, this object relation emerged into consciousness and could be worked with in the treatment.

> Another therapist found herself running several minutes past the appointed end of the session on a routine basis with a particular patient. This was unusual for the therapist, who typically began and ended sessions on time. When the therapist noticed what she was doing and reflected on it, she realized that this patient somehow left her feeling that the therapist was not giving her enough. With this in mind, the therapist became aware of the patient's making similar accusations, always very subtly, in her descriptions of her friends and family members; they never gave the patient what she needed. At this point, the therapist was able to identify the object relation of a frustrated self in interaction with a withholding object, enacted both inside and outside the treatment.

This example illustrates that when a therapist has standard procedures, for example for beginning and ending sessions, it will highlight even minor tendencies on the part of the therapist to behave differently with any particular patient. The therapist's tendency to modify his usual way of working is a form of transference-countertransference enactment. The therapist's recognition that he is tempted or inclined to modify his standard practice with a particular patient provides opportunity to reflect upon, and ultimately to identify and explore, the object relations that are being enacted in the treatment.

THE THERAPEUTIC ALLIANCE

The therapeutic alliance, or treatment alliance, is the working relationship established between the therapist in role, as described above, and the part of the patient that has the capacity for self-observation and holds realistic expectations of receiving and making use of help from the therapist. Thus, the therapeutic alliance is a nonconflictual, positive relationship established between patient and therapist. The quality of the therapeutic alliance has been associated with treatment outcome in a variety of forms of psychotherapy (Horvath and Greenberg 1994; Horvath and Symonds 1991; Orlinsky et al. 1994).

Patients with higher level personality pathology are generally able to establish a stable therapeutic alliance in the early phases of treatment (Gibbons et al. 2003; Marmar et al. 1986; Piper et al. 1991). In DPHP, the development of an alliance is fostered by the structure and reliability of the treatment frame in conjunction with the therapist's interest, understanding, and readiness to listen. For patients who have more difficulty establishing an alliance, early identification and exploration of negative feelings about the therapy and the therapist will help, as will the therapist's maintaining a relatively active stance (Luborsky 1984). (We discuss this process further in discussion of the opening phase of treatment in Chapter 10.) The DPHP therapist does not provide supportive interventions to promote the consolidation of an alliance.

At the same time that the therapeutic alliance is a realistic, helping relationship, it is also based on early transferences to trusted caretakers (Kernberg 2004b). Thus, embedded in the therapeutic alliance is a special form of "benign" positive transference that promotes the progress of the treatment and does not function as a resistance. The benign positive transference as part of the therapeutic alliance can be distinguished from the patient's defensive idealizations of the therapist, which function to avoid anxiety and ward off expression of conflictual motivations in relation to the therapist. In DPHP, idealizing transferences are identified, explored, and interpreted as defending against underlying anxieties. In contrast, the positive transference underlying the treatment alliance is generally left alone and is used to support exploration of the patient's conflictual object relations.

SUGGESTED READINGS

Ackerman S, Hilsenroth M: A review of therapist characteristics and techniques positively impacting the therapeutic alliance. Clin Psychol Rev 23:1–33, 2003

Bender DS: Therapeutic alliance, in The American Psychiatric Publishing Textbook of Personality Disorders. Edited by Oldham JM, Skodol AE, Bender DS. Washington, DC, American Psychiatric Publishing, 2005, pp 405–420

Clarkin JF, Yeomans FE, and Kernberg OF: Assessment phase, II: treatment contracting, in Psychotherapy for Borderline Personality: Focusing on Object Relations. Washington, DC, American Psychiatric Publishing, 2006, pp 209–252

Freud S: Remembering, repeating and working-through (1914), in The Standard Edition of the Complete Psychological Works of Sigmund Freud, Vol 12. Edited and translated by Strachey J. London, Hogarth Press, 1958, pp 147–156

Langs R: The therapeutic relationship and deviations in technique. Int J Psychoanal Psychother 4:106–141, 1975

Martin D, Garske J, Davis M: Relation of the therapeutic alliance with other outcome and other variables: a meta-analytic review. J Consult Clin Psychol 68:438–450, 2000

Samstag LW (ed): Working alliance: current status and future directions. Psychotherapy: Theory, Research, Practice, Training (special edition) 45:257–307, 2006

Sandler J, Dare C, Holder A, et al: Working through, in The Patient and the Analyst, 2nd Edition. Madison, CT, International Universities Press, 1992, pp 121–132

THE TECHNIQUES OF DPHP, PART 1

Listening to the Patient

In this chapter and the chapter that follows, we describe the psychotherapeutic techniques employed by the therapist in dynamic psychotherapy for higher level personality pathology (DPHP). Techniques are the specific methods the therapist uses, moment to moment, when listening to the patient and when making an intervention. In this chapter we describe the techniques involved in the special form of listening that the DPHP therapist employs in his own private thoughts to "hear" the patient's verbal and nonverbal communications. In Chapter 7 we describe the techniques the therapist employs to transform his inner thoughts into verbal interventions that he offers to the patient.

LISTENING TO THE PATIENT

If we were to look at the transcript of a DPHP session, we would be able to discern any number of important issues and conflicts expressed in the material. If we were to look at a videotape of the same session, it is likely that additional issues would present themselves. In DPHP, some issues are introduced in the things the patient says, and others emerge through nonverbal communication. There are issues the patient is aware of bringing into the session, and there are issues that the patient is defending against acknowledging. In DPHP, the therapist opens himself up to receiving as completely as possible the disparate communications provided by the patient, verbally and nonverbally, intentionally and outside his awareness, in any given session.

In DPHP, "listening" to the patient entails not only hearing the content of the patient's words, but also receiving the communications embedded in the patient's behavior and interactions with the therapist. We include here the patient's tone of voice, his body language and facial expressions, his attitude toward the therapist and the treatment, and the discrepancies among these various channels of communication. Listening also entails hearing the patient's associations and the resistances embedded in the material.

When listening to the patient in DPHP, the therapist wants to determine what specific relationship is being enacted in the patient's verbal and nonverbal communications, and also what this relationship is defending against. In considering these questions, the therapist will ask himself, "What is the relationship implicit in the things the patient is telling me today?" "What is the relationship implicit in how she is interacting with me?" "What is the relationship between how the patient is acting and what she is saying?" and "How do the object relations currently enacted relate to previous sessions and recent events in the patient's life?" Throughout this process, the therapist also attends to his own internal reactions to the patient, considering, "How am I feeling toward this patient?" and "How is the patient making me feel today?"

HEARING THE PATIENT'S VERBAL COMMUNICATIONS

LISTENING FOR RELATIONSHIP PATTERNS IN THE PATIENT'S VERBAL COMMUNICATIONS

In DPHP, the treatment setting and the psychotherapeutic relationship tend to activate the patient's conflictual object relations, which are then enacted in the session. Typically, one or two relationship patterns can be seen recurring during a given session. Perhaps the most common way for a patient to bring a particular object relation into the treatment is by describing a particular interpersonal interaction in the course of his open communication with the therapist. Typically the patient will describe an interaction in which he took part, but sometimes the dominant relationship pattern described will not involve the patient directly. Either way, the therapist will assume that the patient is at some level identified with one or both (or, in the case of a triadic relationship pattern, all three) positions in the object relation.

CLINICAL ILLUSTRATION OF LISTENING FOR RELATIONSHIP PATTERNS

A patient described having passed a boy and his father in the street. The father was loudly criticizing the boy in a tone that sounded both hostile and threatening to the patient. The boy seemed hurt and frightened. In describing the scene, the patient commented on his own feelings of wanting to protect the child. The relationship patterns being enacted are of a frightened child in relation to an angry, critical father and of a protective parent in relation to a vulnerable, frightened child. Implicit is a relationship between a child and a parent who does not intervene or protect. In this vignette, the patient is consciously identifying in himself the wish to step in as a third party to protect the child.

Later in the session, the patient described a movie in which a mother repeatedly exposes her children to dangerous situations. The therapist heard once again the relationship pattern of a frightened child exposed to danger who needs, but does not have, a third party to protect him. In this version, the focus is less on the object relation enacted by the father and son in the street, representing the danger, and more on the failure to protect. Listening to the patient, it is clear to the therapist that the patient's description of the movie and of the father and son in the street are bringing the same cluster of object relations into the treatment, and that these relationship patterns are a recurring theme in the session.

WHICH ROLE IS THE PATIENT CONSCIOUSLY IDENTIFIED WITH?

Once the therapist identifies the relationship patterns that appear to be dominant in the patient's verbal communications, the therapist begins to think about which party or parties the patient is currently consciously identified with in any given object relation. In the example above, the patient tells the therapist that he is identified with a protective parent, and he is in addition likely aware of identifying with a parent who fails to protect. It is also possible that the patient is, or can relatively easily become, conscious of his identification with a frightened, endangered, and unprotected child. The patient is probably less aware of his anxiety about his own hostility and sadism, represented both in the image of the father and in the potential dangers to which the children in the movie were exposed.

WHICH ROLE IS THE PATIENT ATTRIBUTING TO THE THERAPIST?

In addition to considering the roles with which the patient is identified, the therapist will also always ask himself, "What are the roles in which the patient is consciously and unconsciously experiencing the therapist?" By keeping this question in mind, the therapist can remain attentive to what is being enacted in the transference, regardless of whether or not the patient directly relates the therapist to the object relations he is describing. When listening to the relationship patterns in the patient's communications, the therapist can ask himself, "How do I fit in?" "How is the patient currently experiencing me?" and "How is the patient currently trying *not* to experience me?" In this particular example, we would wonder, "Is the therapist seen as a protective parent, or perhaps as a parent who exposes the patient to danger without sufficiently protecting him? Is the patient attempting to avoid experiencing the therapist as a hostile, frightening father, or, perhaps, as a frightened, vulnerable child?"

LISTENING TO THE PATIENT'S ASSOCIATIONS

As we have described, in DPHP, it is the patient's role to speak in an unstructured way, as freely and openly as possible, about whatever goes through his mind while in his therapy session. As a patient speaks freely and allows his mind to wander, he will naturally move through thoughts that are linked or associated in his mind. Sometimes these links will be conscious and obvious; at other times, the links between the patient's thoughts will not be apparent to the patient until the therapist points out a connection. We refer to these links as *associations;* by this we mean the connections we can make between seemingly unrelated communications that come to a patient's mind during the course of a therapy session. We can use the patient's associations to learn more about the internal object relations currently activated in the patient's inner world. As the therapist listens, he is always thinking, "What are the different relationship patterns that the patient is describing in this session, and how do they fit together?"

CLINICAL ILLUSTRATIONS OF LISTENING TO THE PATIENT'S ASSOCIATIONS

A young professional woman presented to treatment with marital difficulties. In a session 2 months into the treatment, the patient complained about her husband, who seemed totally preoccupied with work. When he came home, he barely seemed to notice her or the nice dinners she prepared. The patient felt that he did not even really care whether or not she was there; he just wanted to focus on his e-mail.

Later in the session, the patient described a recent family gathering. As always, her mother paid attention to the patient's younger sister while the patient felt ignored. Mother seemed oblivious to all the efforts the patient had made to plan this family get-together. The therapist heard the two anecdotes, about the husband and the mother, as associations, linked and representing the same object relation. On the basis of the patient's associations, the therapist suggested to the patient that in her difficulties with her husband, it seemed that she was feeling like a neglected child, trying to please and get attention from a distracted mother who was too preoccupied with other things to notice her. Although the patient had not been aware of a link between her feelings in relation to her husband and her lifelong diffi-culties with her mother, as soon as the therapist pointed this out, it made sense to her.

Another patient presented to treatment with inhibitions relating to profes-sional success. The patient came into a session, filled with excitement, to tell his therapist that he had been offered a long hoped-for promotion. The patient enjoyed his good fortune for several minutes in the session, then went on to talk about other things. Listening, the therapist realized that the patient had begun talking about a series of misfortunes that had beset peo-ple whom the patient cared about; the patient reported that his brother's son was ill and that his roommate's fiancée had broken off their engage-ment. Next, the patient found himself thinking about the day, 4 years ear-lier, that his sister's application to law school had been rejected. In continuing to listen to the patient's associations, the therapist inferred a linkage between a self that was successful and excited and an object that was defeated, hurt, or unfortunate. This latter relationship pattern was con-nected with feelings of sadness and guilt in relation to success.

"HEARING" THE PATIENT'S NONVERBAL COMMUNICATIONS

In a DPHP session, patient and therapist are always interacting; the patient is always saying or doing something, and the therapist is always responding to the patient—sometimes visibly and at other times internally; sometimes verbally and also nonverbally. The ongoing interaction between therapist and patient is associated with emotional reactions on the part of both par-ticipants. The DPHP therapist wants to open himself up as much as possi-ble to the impact of the patient's verbal and nonverbal communications, allowing the patient to affect him internally.

In this process, the therapist identifies, transiently, with the patient's subjective experience and with the patient's currently enacted internal ob-jects. The therapist then stands back and reflects on his own inner experi-ence of interacting with the patient. Alternating between these two stances in relation to the patient and his interactions with the patient, the therapist establishes himself as a "participant-observer" in the session.

We assume that the feelings induced in the therapist by the patient's words and his behavior reflect conscious and unconscious communications from the patient. Although the therapist's internal responses to the patient's communi-cations always reflect aspects of the therapist's needs, the therapist's responses will also reflect the patient's needs, as well as the therapist's responses to them. With all this in mind, the therapist "listens" and then reflects on what he can learn about the patient from his own internal reactions to him. With a reasonable amount of clinical experience and supervision, most therapists learn to sort through and make use of their reactions to the patient as a channel through which the therapist can "hear" many of the issues raised in a session. The therapist's capacity to make full use of his internal reactions to the patient can be enhanced by the therapist's own experience as a patient in psychotherapy.

MAKING USE OF COUNTERTRANSFERENCE

Implicit in the therapist's stance as participant observer is recognition of the importance of the therapist's countertransference. We use the term *countertransference* in the broad sense, to include all of the therapist's emotional responses to the patient (Kernberg 1975). When the term is used in this way, the countertransference will be codetermined by 1) the patient's transferences to the therapist, 2) the patient's life situation, 3) the therapist's transferences to the patient, and 4) the therapist's life situation. In DPHP, it is assumed that the therapist has a steady flow of emotional reactions to the patient. It is the job of the DPHP therapist to constantly monitor his own countertransference.

In DPHP, the feelings the patient elicits in the therapist are equal in importance to anything the patient may communicate in words about his current internal situation. This is because one of the many ways in which patients defend themselves in DPHP is by inducing attitudes and feelings in the therapist. For example, a patient afraid of erotic feelings might induce irritation, withdrawal, or boredom on the part of the therapist. A patient afraid of being criticized may be extremely ingratiating or behave in ways that are pleasing to the therapist. Alternatively, a patient afraid of his anger might induce feelings of irritation or even anger in the therapist while remaining calm himself, or a patient afraid of his erotic desires might behave in a seductive manner without realizing he is doing so. In each of these situations, the patient is eliciting a response in the therapist for purposes of reducing his own anxiety.

Patients with higher level personality pathology can affect their therapists in subtle and socially appropriate ways that may be almost imperceptible at first. The patient will generally be unaware of what he is doing, and it may take the therapist some time to catch on as well. As a result, the DPHP therapist always pays careful attention to his reactions to the patient and his behavior in relation to the patient, and he tries to understand both in terms of the dominant object relations currently being enacted in the treatment. Early in treatment, the feelings that patients induce in their therapists are typically expressions of a defensive object relationship, along the lines of those induced by the patients who were sexually inhibited or afraid of being criticized, as described above. Later in treatment, we are more likely to see the patient inducing feelings in the therapist that are a more direct expression of the object relation being defended against—for example, the patient who induces anger in his therapist while remaining unaware of angry feelings of his own, or the patient who behaves seductively without realizing he is doing so. Countertransferences of this kind call upon the therapist to tolerate identifying with the patient when he is under the control of conflictual, aggressive, sexual, and dependent motivations.

In order to make use of the countertransference, the DPHP therapist allows the patient to "move" him internally, stimulating affects and internal representations that are part of the steady flow of enactments that characterize the treatment. In any given session and moment to moment within the session, the DPHP therapist will transiently identify with the patient's self representation or with the object representations that are being enacted in the treatment, in the service of deepening his understanding of the patient's conflicts. In the moment, the therapist allows himself to feel invested in and empathically attuned to one aspect of the patient's inner world in relation to another.

CONCORDANT AND COMPLEMENTARY IDENTIFICATIONS IN THE COUNTERTRANSFERENCE

From this perspective, the therapist's countertransference can be classified as either "concordant identification in the countertransference" or "complementary identification in the countertransference" (Racker 1957). Concordant identifications in the countertransference involve the therapist's identifying with the current subjective affective experience of the patient, which is to say, with those parts of the patient's internal object world that the patient is presently experiencing as parts of himself. When countertransference is concordant, the therapist's internal experience parallels that of the patient. For example, if a patient says, "I can't find one of the earrings from my grandmother that my mother gave me," the therapist might feel sad. This would represent a concordant countertransference, in which case the therapist might say, "It sounds like your inability to find your grandmother's earring has stirred up feelings of loss."

When identifications in the countertransference are complementary, the therapist identifies with the self or object representation that is paired with the representation with which the patient is currently identified—if the patient is consciously identified with a self representation, the therapist identifies with the corresponding object representation, while if the patient identifies with an object representation, the therapist identifies with the patient's self representation. Complementary identifications typically provide information about aspects of the patient's current subjective experience that he is experiencing as coming toward him from outside of himself rather than emerging from within him. Returning to our example of the patient who cannot find her earring, as he listens to the patient, the therapist might feel critical. In this case, the therapist might say, "I wonder if you are concerned that your mother will be angry or critical that you lost the earring," or, "I wonder if you aren't afraid that I might be critical of you for losing one of the earrings your mother gave you."

As a consequence of concordant identification, the therapist identifies with the patient's central subjective experience. This is the source of ordinary *empathy*, in which the therapist is able to put himself "in the patient's shoes" and imagine feeling what the patient is consciously experiencing. In contrast, under conditions of complementary identification, the therapist identifies with the patient's objects. As a result, in the case of complementary identifications, the therapist is empathizing with aspects of the patient's experience that are currently dissociated, repressed, or projected. Thus, the total empathy of the therapist is with *both* the patient's subjective experience *and* what the patient cannot tolerate experiencing. This view of the therapist's empathy exceeds ordinary empathy in the social sense.

COUNTERTRANSFERENCE MAY REFLECT THE THERAPIST'S NEEDS AND CONFLICTS

The sources of countertransference are the patient's transference to the therapist, the patient's life situation, the therapist's transferences to the patient, and the therapist's life situation. As a result, as the DPHP therapist monitors his reactions to the patient, he also maintains an open attitude toward exploring the source of his reactions. Specifically, the therapist will always be asking himself to what degree his reactions to the patient provide data about the patient's inner world and to what degree they say more about the therapist's current needs and conflicts than they do about the patient's. The need to be open in this way becomes especially clear when a patient comments on the therapist's behavior.

For example, patients not uncommonly will make statements such as "I can see that you are angry" or "You look tired today." At these moments, it is important that the therapist consider what the patient's perception may say about *both* the therapist's current emotional situation *and* the patient's, rather than simply focusing on one or the other. If the patient's observation is an accurate perception, it is helpful for the therapist to acknowledge this straightforwardly, while refraining from offering explanation or apology. The honest acknowledgment of a shared reality helps to maintain a realistic treatment alliance between therapist and patient. However, once a shared reality has been acknowledged, the therapist should help the patient explore his experience of his interaction with the therapist.

For example, if the patient notices that the therapist has become sleepy during a session and comments on this, the therapist might respond, "You are right, I did feel sleepy. What are your thoughts, what does it mean to you that I became sleepy?" An intervention of this kind is not easy to make without becoming defensive, and dealing in this way with one's own partial acting out requires a high degree of professional responsibility and honesty. Beyond acknowledging the accuracy of the patient's perceptions, we generally do not recommend further self-disclosure on the part of the therapist.

CONTAINING THE COUNTERTRANSFERENCE

In DPHP, many of the therapist's concordant and complementary identifications in the countertransference are both transient and subject to reflection on the part of the therapist. After allowing himself to respond internally to the patient, the DPHP therapist moves into the position of observer. From this vantage point the therapist observes, as a third party, the object relation activated in his own mind in response to his interactions with the patient. It is this process of "triangulation" that enables the therapist to use the countertransference to further his understanding of the object relations currently dominant in the treatment. The capacity to triangulate in this way is the cornerstone of what is referred to as *containment* (Bion 1962a).

Containment is a complex process that can be thought of as taking place in several steps, although in practice the steps we describe may be superimposed on one another. In the most general sense, containment refers to the capacity of thought and self-reflection to modify mental contents, especially highly affectively charged mental contents. Containment implies the capacity to fully experience an emotion without being controlled by that experience or having to turn immediately to action; containment implies both emotional freedom and self-awareness. In psychotherapy, containment always follows upon an interaction between therapist and patient in which the patient affects the therapist internally, stimulating affects and activating representations of self and others in the therapist's inner world.

Next, the "containing" therapist moves into the role of observer and reflects on what has been stimulated in him in his interaction with the patient. Finally, the therapist makes use of the experience to make inferences about the internal object relations being activated in the patient and enacted in the treatment. In this process, the therapist "contains," and in some way modifies, the internal experience stimulated in him by the patient.

Containment enables the therapist to make use of the countertransference as a valuable source of information about the object relations currently being enacted in the treatment, and it allows the therapist to empathize with all parts of the patient and with all sides of any given conflict. Containment calls on the therapist to be both responsive and restrained. The "containing" therapist needs to have the emotional freedom to respond internally to the patient, along with the restraint to delay acting on these responses until he has had opportunity to reflect on them. Another way to say this is that the containing therapist is internally responsive but not interpersonally reactive, replacing action and reaction with self-observation and reflection. Containment may lead to interpretation, but it need not necessarily do so.

CLINICAL ILLUSTRATION OF MAKING USE OF COUNTERTRANSFERENCE

The patient was a 45-year-old single professional woman with no children. She spoke at great length about her wonderful weekend with her boyfriend, focusing on the great sex and the great fun, the colorful people, the beautiful homes. As the session progressed, the patient became more and more excited. Her tone became shrill; she spoke and laughed loudly as she told humorous stories in an extremely animated fashion.

Initially, the female therapist (several years younger than her patient) was swept up in the patient's mood, feeling excited herself and wanting to laugh along with the patient. (This is an example of concordant identification in the countertransference.) However, as she continued to sit with the patient, she started to feel diminished and demoralized, and she found herself thinking that the patient had things the therapist would never have. (This is a complementary identification in the countertransference.)

Reflecting on her own responses to the patient's verbal and nonverbal communications, the therapist identified an object relation of an excited person who "has it all" and an excluded and inferior person who feels envious. Thinking about it further, the therapist was struck by how exaggeratedly diminished she had been feeling. She remembered the envy the patient had felt in the past toward the therapist, whom the patient knew was married and had children.

As the therapist reflected on what was being enacted in the session and why, the therapist found herself feeling calmer in the face of the patient's manic style, and she was able to empathize with the painful feelings underlying the patient's excitement. As the session went on, the patient, too, began to calm somewhat and became more self-reflective.

FAILURES OF CONTAINMENT

The therapist's capacity to contain the countertransference distinguishes countertransference that serves as a vehicle for understanding the patient's inner world from countertransference that acts as a vehicle for limiting or even disrupting the therapeutic process. Further, there are times when the therapist's capacity to contain the patient's affects in the countertransference may be a therapeutic intervention in and of itself. In contrast, when a therapist is chronically unable to contain a particular countertransference and is, further, unable to reflect upon failures of containment, countertransference can put constraints on the therapist's capacity to understand the patient's internal situation.

In particular, subtle but chronic countertransference enactments, often expressed in the therapist's maintaining a particular attitude toward or feeling about a patient over time, can be difficult for the therapist to diagnose. Common examples are patients we tend to see as in some way special—for example, as particularly needy or vulnerable or desirable. Chronic countertransferences of this kind are typically ego syntonic for the therapist, and for the patient as well. As a result, chronic countertransference reactions may be enacted for extended periods of time without being noticed by the therapist. Unexamined countertransferences, both acute and chronic, cause blind spots in the therapist and will make it difficult for him to understand or empathize with particular aspects of the patient's conscious and unconscious experience.

CLINICAL ILLUSTRATION OF FAILURES OF CONTAINMENT

Let's return to the vignette of the 45-year-old single woman discussed above. The patient stimulated in the therapist feelings first of excitement and then of diminishment. If the therapist had failed to contain her responses to the patient, she might have joined the patient in manic excitement, identifying with the patient's conscious self representation and denying the painful object relation that was being split off. In this situation, the therapist would be colluding with the patient's defensive efforts to avoid awareness of underlying object relations. Alternatively, the therapist might have gotten lost in her own feelings of envy and demoralization, allowing them to interfere with her capacity to reflect on how and why she felt this way in relation to the patient. This could leave the therapist with a blind spot, unable to empathize with the patient's underlying feelings of envy and inferiority, and might lead the therapist to withdraw from the patient.

We can also use this patient and her therapist to illustrate failures of containment of *chronic* countertransference reactions. We will at this point add that this particular patient was quite an impressive individual. She was extremely successful professionally in a high-profile and highly influential position. Further, she was very attractive physically and was always elegantly dressed. The therapist had great admiration for the things the patient had accomplished, as well as for how attractively she presented herself. It was only after the patient had been in treatment for almost a year that the therapist became fully aware of the subtle way in which her admiration for the patient limited her capacity to fully empathize with the part of the patient that felt small, left out, and sad. As is typical of more subtle, chronic countertransference reactions, the therapist's implicit attitude toward the patient enacted an object relation that was both familiar to and ego syntonic for the patient and the therapist alike, and it was therefore easy for the therapist's attitude to go largely unnoticed for a long time.

Although the therapist's attitude had been fully conscious, it had not been fully acknowledged or explored. It was only after the treatment had deepened and the patient began to openly reveal her chronic, underlying sense of sadness and isolation that the therapist fully appreciated the impact that her own attitude toward the patient had had on her capacity to empathize with the patient's internal situation.

TOLERATING UNCERTAINTY

An intrinsic component of the DPHP therapist's capacity to listen to and to hear his patient is his capacity to tolerate uncertainty. It may not be clear in a given session, or at times even over the course of several sessions, which issue is the dominant one in the treatment or what is going on in the transference-countertransference. It often takes time for things to crystallize, and some degree of uncertainty on the part of the therapist, much of the time, is to be expected.

The feeling of not knowing can generate anxiety—especially in the less experienced therapist, who may feel that someone more skilled would have a clearer understanding of what is going on. This rather expectable anxiety should be contained as well as possible. To this end, it can be helpful for the therapist to remind himself that expecting to always understand what is going on is an unreasonable demand to place on himself. At the same time, the therapist should consider whether there is something going on in the patient or in the countertransference that is leaving the therapist particularly anxious to "know" what is happening. It is preferable to wait and see what comes of uncertainty, as well as to consider whether there may be specific meaning to the uncertainty or confusion experienced in a session, rather than to make a premature formulation as an effort to make uncertainty and anxiety go away. It is fine for the therapist to acknowledge to the patient at times that he is not yet clear about what is happening and that a clearer understanding will emerge with time.

If a therapist is rarely uncertain, it probably reflects that he is approaching the material with preconceived ideas about what is going on and that he is hearing what the patient has to say with an ear toward having it conform to his own expectations. Even if it is relatively subtle, the therapist's inability to tolerate not knowing, with a propensity to hear the patient's communications as a validation of what the therapist "already knows," is a form of countertransference acting out, often tied to an excessive allegiance on the part of the therapist to a particular theory. While theory will always unconsciously inform and to some degree direct our listening, we should do everything possible to maintain an open mind.

SUGGESTED READINGS

Britton R: Naming and containing, in Belief and Imagination. London, Routledge, 1998, pp 19–28

Busch F: Free association, in The Ego at the Center of Analytic Technique. Northvale, NJ, Jason Aronson, 1995, pp 49–70

Kernberg OF: Acute and chronic countertransference reactions, in Aggressivity, Narcissism and Self-Destructiveness in the Psychotherapeutic Relationship. New Haven, CT, Yale University Press, 2004, pp 167–183

Langs R: Therapeutic misalliances. Int J Psychoanal Psychother 4:77–105, 1975

Lowenstein RM: Some considerations on free association. J Am Psychoanal Assoc 11:451–473, 1963

Ogden TH: The concept of projective identification (1982), in Projective Identification and Psychotherapeutic Technique. Northvale, NJ, Jason Aronson, 1993, pp 11–38

Racker H: The meanings and uses of countertransference. Psychoanal Q 26:303–357, 1957

Sandler J, Sandler AM: On role-responsiveness, in Internal Objects Revisited. London, International Universities Press, 1998, pp 47–56

7

THE TECHNIQUES OF DPHP, PART 2

Intervening

We have described the techniques the therapist uses in dynamic psycho-therapy for higher level personality pathology (DPHP) to listen to and understand his patient's verbal and nonverbal communications. After lis-tening, the therapist will formulate an intervention. In DPHP, the major verbal interventions made by the therapist involve analysis of resistance and interpretation of unconscious conflict. When making verbal interventions, the therapist attempts to intervene from a position of technical neutrality.

TECHNICAL NEUTRALITY

When we say that the DPHP therapist maintains "technical neutrality," we mean that the therapist avoids using supportive techniques and avoids taking sides in the patient's conflicts. Supportive techniques commonly employed in psychotherapy include offering advice, teaching coping skills, and directly intervening in the patient's life. "Not taking sides" means that the therapist refrains from speaking for one side of a patient's conflict in relation to the others.

In contrast to DPHP, many forms of dynamic psychotherapy employ a combination of supportive and expressive techniques, and the therapist does not maintain a neutral stance (Gabbard 2004). In these treatments, the therapist employs supportive techniques on a "sliding scale," depending on the clinical needs of the patient at any particular point in the treatment. However, in our experience, it is preferable to make a distinction between the techniques of supportive (Rockland 1989) and exploratory psychotherapy and to restrict the use of supportive interventions when exploratory therapy is prescribed. In DPHP, technical neutrality facilitates the activation of conflictual internal object relations in the treatment and enhances the therapist's capacity to effectively explore and interpret the expressive and defensive relationship patterns enacted in the treatment.

DEFINING TECHNICAL NEUTRALITY

At the same time that technical neutrality is central to the technique of DPHP, it is a problematic and controversial construct that must be used flexibly if it is to be integrated into a dynamic understanding of the complex interactions and steady flow of enactments that take place between patient and therapist. Our general approach with regard to maintaining technical neutrality is that the therapist formulates his verbal interventions from a technically neutral position, exercises restraint in his interactions with the patient, monitors the countertransference, and maintains an awareness that in the microprocess of his interactions with the patient, there will be a steady flow of enactments that he will participate in more or less actively.

From a theoretical perspective, technical neutrality implies that the therapist maintains a stance that avoids siding with any one of the conflicting motivations within the patient (Apfelbaum 2005; Moore and Fine 1995). Rather than becoming involved in the patient's conflicts, the neutral therapist is interested in helping the patient to identify and explore his conflicts and to do so evenhandedly, from a variety of perspectives (Levy and Inderbitzin 1992). Because psychological conflicts are organized around internal object relations, neutrality implies that the therapist abstains from supporting or rejecting motivations associated with conflictual self and object representations activated in the patient's internal world. For example, if a patient is complaining about how unfair or controlling his boss is, the neutral therapist would abstain from either castigating the boss or pointing out to the patient how he is being unfair, but instead would try to clarify the object relation being enacted in the patient's interactions with his boss.

Technical neutrality calls upon the therapist to be open to as broad an array of conflicting motivations and anxieties within the patient as is possible, while maintaining an attitude that is accepting, nonjudgmental, and nonpartisan (Schafer 1983). Rather than becoming invested in or rejecting of the motives or attitudes associated with one or another of the patient's conflictual internal object relations, or supporting the demands of reality, the neutral therapist allies himself with the part of the patient that has a capacity for self-observation. Over time, this alliance will help fortify the patient's capacity for self-observation and self reflection (Kernberg 2004b). The neutral therapist and the self-observing part of the patient work together, with the shared goal of understanding the patient's inner life and subjective experience as completely as possible.

TECHNICAL NEUTRALITY AND SOCIAL EXPECTATIONS

Establishing and maintaining technical neutrality means that the DPHP therapist adopts and maintains a stance in relation to the patient's communications and conflicts that is different from that taken by any other person in the patient's life. Typically, when listening to someone discuss a problem, we will think in terms of "How can I make this person feel better?" or "How can I help him solve this problem?" or "Is this person doing the right thing?" In contrast, the neutral therapist will think, "How can I most completely understand what this patient is saying and doing?" This deviation from social norms can seem odd or feel uncomfortable for the patient, especially early in treatment, and it may also be uncomfortable for therapists at times, particularly therapists who have not had much experience with working with patients in this way.

It can be helpful to keep in mind that recommending DPHP to a patient implies that the therapist believes DPHP is the most effective way to alleviate the patient's suffering. If DPHP is the treatment of choice, it follows that it is in the best interest of the patient for the therapist to adhere to the technique of DPHP, giving the patient opportunity to benefit as fully as possible from all that DPHP has to offer. In this sense, maintaining technical neutrality is an expression of concern for the patient on the part of the therapist. When a DPHP therapist abstains from offering the kind of support or advice that a patient desires at a given moment, he does so with the expectation that a neutral stance is what will be most helpful to the patient in the long run.

QUALITY OF INTERACTIONS BETWEEN
NEUTRAL THERAPIST AND PATIENT

The term *neutrality* can raise concern that we are suggesting that the DPHP therapist assume an attitude of relative indifference in relation to the patient or that he attempt to conceal his personality and adopt a bland stance when in his professional role. This is decidedly not true. When we speak of "neutrality," we are not referring to the therapist's attitude toward the patient or to his interpersonal behavior in relation to the patient. Rather, "technical neutrality" refers to the therapist's attitude toward the patient's internal conflicts.

Technical neutrality does not imply that the therapist is unresponsive in his interactions with the patient, nor does it imply that the therapist is indifferent to the patient's progress. Rather, the DPHP therapist should be responsive and genuine, rather than stiff or robotic, and his attitude toward the patient should reflect concern for the patient and for the patient's well-being. The neutral therapist maintains a professional attitude that communicates warmth and concern while being respectful of the patient's autonomy. At the same time, it is also true that, while a DPHP therapist needs to be emotionally responsive to his patient, a therapist who is excessively responsive or solicitous is likely to encroach on the patient's freedom to explore conflicts activated in the treatment as completely as might otherwise be possible.

What we suggest is that the therapist be responsive but also restrained in his attitude and behavior in relation to the patient. DPHP cannot be effective if the therapist is routinely acting on and communicating his own needs in the patient's treatment. In the end, a patient will be able to sense whether or not the therapist is genuinely concerned for the patient's well-being and genuinely committed to putting his own needs aside for the benefit of the patient's treatment. When the patient feels that these things are not true, the treatment is not a "safe" place for the patient to explore his inner world.

CLINICAL ILLUSTRATION OF TECHNICAL NEUTRALITY

As a relatively simple example of a therapist's maintaining a neutral stance, consider the patient who complains, apparently justifiably, about his wife's critical and withholding nature. In so doing, the patient is describing a self representation and an object representation. A neutral therapist does not side with the patient's self experience—for example, by expressing sympathy for the patient or criticism of the patient's wife. Neither does the neutral therapist side with the patient's object representation—for example, by pointing out to the patient that he is being unfair or unkind to his wife. Neither will the therapist side with the demands of reality, by counseling the patient as to the best way to handle his wife or by trying to figure out who is at fault.

Rather, a neutral therapist will listen to the patient's description and complaints with his ear tuned toward the following questions:

- "What does this tell me about the patient's inner experience and the internal object relations active in the treatment at this moment?"
- "What object relation is the patient playing out with his wife?"

- "What object relation is the patient playing out with me in complaining about his wife?"
- "What object relation is the patient defending against in his interactions with his wife and with me?"

DEVIATIONS FROM TECHNICAL NEUTRALITY

Deviations from neutrality, if chronic and not openly addressed, can interfere with the full emergence of the patient's conflicts in the treatment and will make it less likely that they can be worked through in the transference. In essence, by consistently siding with particular self or object representation or with the defensive or expressive side of a conflict, the therapist is actively playing a role in or acting out an aspect of the patient's inner world in the relationship between patient and therapist. Enactments of this kind tend to be resistant to interpretation and, at the same time, may preclude other object relations from emerging in the treatment. Similarly, if the therapist actively sides with or speaks for the parts of the patient motivated to meet the demands of reality as effectively as possible, the therapist may drive underground those parts of the patient that are motivated to do otherwise.

As an example of a deviation from neutrality, imagine that the therapist is actively and routinely supportive of the patient described above and is critical of the patient's wife. In this situation, the therapist's "support" of the patient (and in this process, of the patient's defenses) may make it more difficult for the patient to gain awareness that, in his own critical attitude toward his wife, he is himself identifying with the critical and withholding object representation that he has been experiencing in relation to his wife (a form of role reversal). A deviation from neutrality of this kind might also shut down an opportunity for the conflicts with the wife to be activated in the transference. In contrast, if the therapist is neutral, the patient will have room to wonder if the therapist may also be critical of him or withholding of love and support, or he may find himself feeling critical of the therapist. Exploration of these questions will further open up the internal object relations and self and object representations active in the patient's conflicts with his wife.

In sum, deviations from neutrality can interfere with full emergence of all sides of the patient's conflicts into consciousness and will also make it less likely that they can be worked with in the transference. Chronic or unnoticed deviations on the part of the therapist can lead to a therapeutic impasse.

CLINICAL ILLUSTRATION OF ESTABLISHING A NEUTRAL STANCE AT THE BEGINNING OF TREATMENT

As an example of how and why the DPHP therapist establishes a neutral stance at the beginning of treatment, let us return to the 34-year-old, professional woman, discussed in Chapter 5 ("The Strategies of DPHP and the Treatment Setting"), who was stuck in a frustrating relationship with a male colleague. At the point that she came for a consultation and began in treatment, the patient understood that the relationship was not good for her and was most likely going nowhere, but she nevertheless felt unable to leave. Her friends were urging her to give up on this man and move on, but she could not follow their good advice. Other men had approached her, but she found them uninteresting.

If, at the outset, the therapist does not maintain technical neutrality and instead chooses to assume a supportive stance, he might approach this situation in terms of "How can I get the patient to leave this relationship?" In assuming this attitude, the therapist would be siding with the part of the patient that wants to leave, as well as with the demands presented by the reality that she is 34 years old and wants to get married and have a family. Taking this approach, the therapist might impress upon the patient, as have many others, that this man is only frustrating her—she knows he will not marry her—and that continuing to pursue him may compromise her chances of getting married and having a family.

It is possible that the non-neutral therapist could use his authority to pry the patient out of a bad relationship. The problem, however, is that this approach will not give the patient opportunity to understand why she is in the relationship in the first place, nor will it leave her any less likely to re-create the same situation again in the future. The non-neutral or "supportive" therapist may succeed in getting the patient to leave the boyfriend, but he or she is less likely to help the patient solve her underlying problem.

In contrast to the non-neutral therapist who thinks, "How can I get her out?," the DPHP therapist thinks, "How can I understand the fact that she stays?" A neutral stance will focus on uncovering and exploring, as completely as possible, the conflictual object relations embedded in and defended against by the patient's relationship with this man. As these conflicts are worked through, the patient will obtain greater flexibility and freedom to choose whether or not to continue to pursue this man and whether or not to choose a different kind of man in the future.

In the initial phases of the treatment, the neutral DPHP therapist would help this patient become aware that there is a division within her. Part of her, supported by her friends, wants to leave the relationship and move on. Another part wants to pursue this man and continues to be drawn to him. The therapist will help the patient become interested in understanding this conflict and will at the same time abstain from pressuring the patient either to leave or to stay. In so doing, the therapist is not taking sides in the patient's conflict and is at the same time supporting the patient's capacity for self-observation. This will facilitate the patient's bringing the conflictual object relations underlying her romantic difficulties into the treatment.

In contrast, when the supportive therapist condemns the patient's boyfriend and encourages her to give up on the relationship, the therapist is speaking for and siding with one part of the patient against another. Rather than supporting the patient's capacity for self-observation, the supportive therapist's stance actively supports repression and dissociation of the object relations that draw the patient to this man. While this may leave the patient acutely less conflicted and anxious, it does so at the price of making it less likely that, in the end, she will have the opportunity to understand the complex motivations that underlie her romantic choices.

INTERPRETATION

Interpretation and working through of unconscious conflict, in conjunction with analysis of resistance, are the major verbal therapeutic interventions made in DPHP. Interpretations bring to the patient's conscious awareness a conflictual object relation that is being activated and either experienced unconsciously—enacted outside the patient's awareness—or expressed in symptoms. In addition, interpretations make connections or shed light on material against which the patient may be struggling or that the patient may be avoiding.

The process of interpretation will begin from observation of omissions, discrepancies, or contradictions in what the patient is saying and doing, and will lead to explicit hypotheses about these observations so that sense can be made of them. Analysis of resistance involves exploring and interpreting the patient's defensive operations as they are enacted in the treatment. Working through involves a series of interpretations in which a particular conflict is repeatedly experienced and interpreted from various perspectives and in a variety of contexts over a period of time. As previously noted, in DPHP, interpretations are made from a position of technical neutrality.

THE INTERPRETIVE PROCESS

Interpretation is best thought of as a *process* (Sandler et al. 1992). Early steps in the interpretive process typically involve clarification and confrontation. *Clarification* involves the therapist's seeking clarification of the patient's subjective experience. Areas of vagueness are addressed until both the patient and the therapist have a clear understanding of what has been said, or until the patient feels puzzled by an underlying contradiction in his thinking that has been brought to light.

In addition to pointing to aspects of mental experience that have been repressed, clarification often functions to bring to the patient's attention aspects of his subjective experience that, though accessible to consciousness, have been dissociated, denied, or disavowed. In this way, clarification calls the patient's attention to aspects of his subjective experience that he has avoided paying attention to or thinking about. The process of clarification leads very naturally to *confrontation*, which involves the therapist's pulling together clarified information that is contradictory, conflictual, or does not fit together, and then presenting the patient with the material that needs further exploration and understanding. In confrontation, the therapist calls the patient's attention to an area of conflict and defense, in this process focusing and deepening ongoing inquiry.

We hope it is clear that the word *confrontation* is used here as one would speak of being "confronted by a painful reality." "Confrontation" is not used as it would be in a military or political setting to suggest an aggressive clashing of forces. Rather, confrontation involves the therapist's tactfully and thoughtfully pointing out aspects of the patient's verbal and nonverbal communications that bear further consideration. Confrontation may involve addressing discrepancies between the patient's verbal communications in sessions and information the therapist has already been told in previous sessions. Confrontations may also focus on discrepancies between the patient's verbal and nonverbal communications—for example, when a patient discusses painful material in a light, casual tone.

Interpretation proper follows and builds upon clarification and confrontation. Interpretation involves making a link between the patient's conscious, observed behavior, his thoughts and feelings, and the unconscious factors that may be underlying them. In essence, when the therapist offers an interpretation he is presenting the patient with a hypothesis about unconscious or dissociated psychological conflicts that may explain aspects of the patient's words and behaviors that on the surface appear illogical or maladaptive. The aim of an interpretation is to make sense of aspects of the patient's experience and behavior and in this process to deepen the patient's understanding of his inner life. A "complete" interpretation would describe the defense, the anxiety motivating the defense, and the underlying wish, need, or fear being defended against, with each of these three elements described as an internal object relation. However, as we have said, interpretation is a process, and interpretations are typically offered in pieces, giving the patient opportunity to assimilate the therapist's interventions in a stepwise fashion.

CLINICAL ILLUSTRATION OF INTERPRETATION

A middle-aged businessman, in treatment for 6 months, told a story about his business partner's having lied to him. To the therapist, it was clear that the patient was critical of and angry with his partner, but it appeared that the patient was either unaware of or preferred not to acknowledge having angry feelings. The therapist asked the patient about his feelings about his partner's behavior (*clarification*). The patient persisted in not acknowledging negative feelings.

In formulating an interpretation of this conflict, the therapist might say to the patient: "I am struck by the absence of anger or criticism as you describe the situation with your partner. It would only be natural to have such feelings, yet it is as though you try to avoid them" (*confrontation*). The therapist might then pause to clarify whether this was something that the patient understood. If the patient appreciated that his anger was noticeably absent, the therapist might go on to suggest a possible motivation for the patient's behavior. For example, the therapist might say something like, "Could it be that you avoid negative feelings because you fear that they can lead other people to withdraw, and that you avoid feeling critical of your partner because you worry that this would cause him to pull away or even to end your partnership?"

In his interpretation, the therapist began by confronting a contradiction—it would be natural to be angry, but the patient was not. He then went on to describe the patient's motivation for defense, experienced as an anxiety and represented as an internal object relation of a critical self who fears loss of love, and an object who responds to criticism or anger by withdrawing. The conflictual motivations were the patient's anger and wish to criticize, which remained largely out of awareness.

When making an interpretation, a therapist is aware that an object relation described in an initial intervention also serves to defend against enactment of the complementary object relation—that is, the same object relation with the roles reversed. (For example, we might ultimately see enactment of an internal object relation of an angry object in relation to a withdrawing self.) The final steps in any interpretive process involve being able to uncover these links. However, because of the rigidity of defensive operations in higher level personality pathology, it may be quite some time before the patient's identification with the object representation can be made.[1]

In fact, it is not uncommon for the therapist to move on to explore and interpret other underlying conflicts, pointing out how the original object relation defends against activation of these conflicts, before returning to earlier interpretations, now with the roles inverted. However, in the end, in order for a patient to successfully integrate a conflictual object relation into his conscious sense of self, he will need to come to tolerate his identification with both sides of that object relation. Typically, helping the patient work through the conflict as it was originally formulated, along with providing the opportunity to work through other related conflicts, helps the patient tolerate awareness of his identification with what was originally attributed to an object representation.

INTERPRETING FROM SURFACE TO DEPTH

In general, the most tactful way to formulate an interpretation is to begin by addressing the defense and the patient's motivation for defense, and,

---

[1]This is very different from the situation in the treatment of patients with more severe personality pathology, in which the patient typically shifts back and forth between identifying with both halves of an object relation, and interpretation of one object relation as defending against its inverse is usually made quite quickly.

only after having done so, to address the underlying conflictual motivation the patient is defending against. This approach to interpretation is sometimes referred to as the *dynamic principle* of interpretation (Fenichel 1941). The dynamic principle directs the therapist to interpret by beginning with material that serves defensive functions and moving toward material that is defended against. Because object relations serving defensive functions will be closest to consciousness while object relations that are being defended against will be further from the conscious "surface," this approach is sometimes referred to in terms of interpreting "from surface to depth."

In keeping with the dynamic principle, in our example, the therapist began his interpretation by pointing out that the patient seemed to be avoiding negative feelings. The therapist quickly linked this observation to a hypothesis about a motivation for this defensive avoidance—namely, that the patient was afraid that negative feelings would lead to social isolation. By linking defense and motivation in this way, the therapist made it less likely that the patient would feel the therapist was criticizing him for "avoiding his anger" or simply accusing the patient of being angry, and more likely that the patient would feel the therapist understood the dilemma he faced.

In the process of identifying the defense and suggesting a motivation for defense, the therapist implicitly pointed out that the patient had angry and critical feelings that he was either repressing or failing to acknowledge. However, the emphasis in the interpretation is on the patient's experience that it is a psychological necessity to avoid his anger. In DPHP we would focus on understanding why it is so important to this patient to avoid angry feelings, and on identifying the various ways the patient goes about avoiding acknowledging anger; the focus of inquiry is not on "uncovering" or highlighting the patient's anger per se (Busch 1995, 1996).

TRANSFERENCE INTERPRETATION

The interpretation described in the previous subsection—identifying defense, anxiety motivating defense, and conflictual motivation—is considered a complete interpretation that does not involve a representation of or reference to the therapist. At another point in the session, or later in the treatment, the therapist might use his understanding of the unconscious conflict activated by the partner's lying to shed light on the patient's behavior toward the therapist. For example, the therapist might notice that when he has to reschedule or cancel sessions, even when changes seem relatively inconvenient for the patient, this patient is always accommodating and excessively gracious. This observation can lead the therapist to realize that, in essence, the same object relation enacted in relation to the partner is being enacted in the transference as well. If he had already made the interpretation about the partner, the therapist would now be well positioned to link this to the relationship with the therapist by making a *transference interpretation.*

Again, the therapist might begin by pointing out that it would be reasonable under the circumstances for the patient to feel irritated, this time with the therapist, and to indicate the similarity to other situations in which the patient had avoided feeling angry. The therapist could proceed by saying something along the lines of "Could it be that you are trying to avoid critical feelings toward me because, in your mind, to have negative feelings toward me runs the risk that I will withdraw or will not want to work with you, much as you fear your critical feelings will lead to your partner's ending the partnership and withdrawing?"

In DPHP, there is a great deal of variation—both across patients and within a given treatment over time—as to the degree to which the patient's internal object relations are enacted in relation to the therapist. For some patients, the relationship with the therapist becomes a major vehicle for expression of the patient's internal world, whereas for many patients, the relationship with the therapist is relatively protected and conflictual object relations are most visibly enacted in relation to others.

RELATIONSHIP BETWEEN TRANSFERENCE AND EXTRATRANSFERENCE INTERPRETATIONS

In DPHP, interpretations are appropriately made both extratransferentially and in the transference. Typically, the same conflict will be repeatedly activated and interpreted in a variety of ways outside the transference, and will also at times be enacted in the transference. In the *working through* process of the therapy, links are made between extratransferential and transferential experiences whenever possible. This process of repeatedly activating and interpreting a conflict, and of linking various representations of a given conflict as it is activated in the patient's current interpersonal relationships and in his relationship with the therapist, will help the patient gain a deeper and more emotionally meaningful experience of his conflicts.

Sometimes while exploring a conflict enacted in the patient's interpersonal life, the therapist may detect that the same conflict is being activated in the transference, but with manifestations that are too subtle to bring up with the patient in a meaningful or convincing fashion. In this situation, we find that if we analyze in detail the conflict as it is enacted outside the transference, it may set the stage for analyzing the same conflict in the transference. The rationale for this is twofold. First, once a patient is alert to a conflict and to the repetitive enactment of specific conflictual and defensive object relations in his interpersonal life, when the therapist turns attention to the transference he is revisiting a familiar pattern, demonstrating that this is happening "here, too." For many patients, this is easier to understand and more palatable than making the treatment relationship the primary focus of inquiry. In addition, the process of clarifying, confronting, and exploring a given conflict as it is enacted outside the transference often serves to stimulate or intensify enactment of the same conflict in the transference.

As a rule, when the same conflict is activated simultaneously in the transference and extratransferentially, we begin interpretation where the conflict is closest to consciousness. If a given object relation is consciously experienced both in relation to the therapist and in relation to others in the patient's life, we begin our exploration in whichever area is invested with the most affect.

INTERPRETATION AND THE PATIENT'S PAST

In DPHP, interpretations are made predominantly in the here and now. This means that most interpretations focus on the patient's current anxieties, as they are activated and experienced in his daily life and in the treatment. At times it will be easy to propose links between current conflictual object relations and important relationships and events in the patient's developmental past. Interpretations of this kind, which make links to the past, are sometimes referred to as *genetic interpretations.*

In the treatment of patients with high-level personality pathology, early or excessive focus on the past, using the patient's presenting, conscious experience of early objects and his developmental history, can lead to an overly intellectual, "pseudo-psychoanalytic" interaction between patient and therapist, to some degree removed from the immediacy of the patient's current affective experience. This will protect the patient from experiencing conflicts in an immediate and affectively meaningful fashion. In addition, excessive or premature use of genetic interpretations can interfere with the emergence of more deeply repressed internal object relations. In contrast, during the later phases of treatment, genetic interpretation can work to further deepen the patient's emotional experience of those conflictual object relations that have already been interpreted and to some degree worked through.

CLINICAL ILLUSTRATION OF MAKING INTERPRETIVE LINKS TO THE DEVELOPMENTAL PAST

As an example of a genetic interpretation, let us return to the man fearful of feeling critical of his partner. In initially portraying his history, the patient described a happy childhood and a loving relationship with both of his parents. However, during the course of treatment, he recounted feelings of painful isolation during latency and early adolescence. He remembered having felt that his father withdrew from him during those years, and having imagined that his own critical feelings had been responsible for his father's withdrawal.

A genetic interpretation might be offered at this point, referring back to the object relation of a critical self and a withdrawing or rejecting partner. The therapist might suggest that perhaps the patient fears that his critical or angry feelings could lead to the painful isolation he felt as a child in relation to his father. In this way, the therapist could make a link between the object relation of a critical self and a withdrawing object, and representations of early experiences with father that had been repressed or disavowed because they were anxiety provoking or painful.

In this example, the patient's childhood fantasy of having driven father away with his own angry criticism defended against a more painful experience of having himself felt helplessly driven away by father's anger. The situation with the partner and with the rescheduling therapist stimulated feelings of anger toward someone upon whom the patient felt dependent, and left him fearful of ending up isolated as a result of his critical feelings. However, beneath these concerns were concerns about being dependent upon someone who could be angry and critical. Here we are pointing out that even when we offer hypotheses about the developmental roots of a patient's current conflicts, we do so knowing that we are not reconstructing historical events that "explain" the patient's current conflicts and personality rigidity. Rather, when we make interpretations in relation to the patient's past, we are creating connections that make sense of one part of a complex picture, connections that will be reworked and revised throughout the course of the treatment.

ANALYSIS OF RESISTANCE

In the natural course of events, a patient's conflictual object relations will be activated in his daily life and in his relationship with the neutral therapist. Once activated, there is a tension between the tendency to enact the conflictual object relations that have been activated and the opposing tendency to further repress or otherwise defend against their direct expression. *Analysis of resistance* refers to the process of exploring and interpreting the patient's defensive operations as they are activated and enacted in the treatment.

RESISTANCE AND ANALYSIS OF DEFENSE

The term *resistance* is used to refer to the patient's defensive operations as they are expressed in therapy (Moore and Fine 1995) because, typically, the patient's defensive operations will be expressed in the form of some sort of resistance to open communication or self-observation. In essence, the patient resists awareness of aspects of his self experience that are conflictual; the presence of resistance reflects the patient's turning to repression, splitting, denial, or disavowal in the face of psychological conflict. What these defensive operations have in common is a sense of "not wanting to see."

The term *resistance* should not be taken to imply that the patient is consciously resisting or intentionally working against the treatment. Resistances, like defensive operations in general, are automatic and largely unconscious, and will typically be invisible to the patient, even if they are quite apparent to the therapist. Resistances are self-protective mechanisms on the part of the patient, and they function to avoid the negative affects of anxiety, guilt, fear, depression, disappointment, loss, and shame that are associated with the activation and enactment of conflictual object relations.

Analysis of resistance refers to the identification, exploration, and, ultimately, interpretation of anxieties and defenses activated in the treatment and enacted in the transference. Analysis of resistance does not imply attacking, pushing through, or plowing over the patient's self-protective mechanisms. Rather, analysis of resistance entails empathizing with the patient's anxiety while exploring and working through the conflictual object relations embedded in his defensive operations.

Patients often experience resistance as something that interferes with or makes it difficult to communicate freely and openly with the therapist. The patient may say that he feels stuck or does not know what to talk about, or he may seem to avoid something, either purposefully or without being aware of what he is doing. He may change subjects or neglect the implications of something he has been talking about. Therapists can identify the presence of a resistance by asking themselves whether anything appears to be interfering with the patient's communicating openly and freely in the session. Are there frequent silences, or is the patient having difficulty deciding what to talk about? If the patient is speaking, are there things apparently being omitted or avoided? If the answer to any of these questions is "Yes," the priority in the session is to explore the patient's conscious and unconscious experience of communicating with the therapist.

RESISTANCE AND INTERPRETATION

Following the general rules of interpretation, the analysis of resistance begins at the surface, with *clarification* of the patient's experience followed by the therapist's pointing out to the patient that something appears to be missing or denied in the patient's verbal communications (*confrontation*). This intervention will be followed by exploration of the motivation for and meaning of the omission. The therapist's approach is first to point out an area of difficulty or apparent avoidance. For example, the therapist might say: "You have told me a great deal about your relationship with your wife, but I notice that you have said nothing about your sexual life" or "You have told me all about what a wonderful mother she has been, but virtually nothing about her limitations." Or the therapist might comment on the patient's style of communication, for example: "I notice that whenever you begin to talk about your ambitions, you seem to hesitate before speaking." Having identified and confronted an area of resistance, the therapist explores with the patient the anxiety underlying his difficulty communicating.

The presence of resistance implies that the patient is warding off anxiety associated with conflicts being activated in the treatment. As resistances are explored, the anxiety the patient is experiencing—or, more accurately, the anxiety the patient is automatically trying to avoid experiencing—will typically be enacted in the transference. For example, the patient who avoids talking about his sexual relationship with his wife may fear that if he were more open, the therapist would not approve of his sexual life, or would want to intrude, or would take prurient pleasure in hearing about other people's sexual practices. With the patient who only speaks favorably of her mother, it may emerge that she believes the therapist disapproves of women who criticize their mothers. The patient who hesitates before acknowledging his ambitions may fear that the therapist would see him as aggressive or greedy if he were open about his aspirations. Each of these anxieties can be described in terms of an object relation that the patient resists experiencing in relation to the therapist. Thus, analysis of resistance can quickly bring the patient's anxieties and defensive operations into the transference.

When analyzing a resistance, we begin by pointing out that something appears to be blocking open communication or self-awareness, and then we go on to suggest that this must be motivated by some sort of anxiety. In essence, we ask the patient: "If you were to speak openly and freely here about the aspect of your inner experience that you seem to be avoiding, forgetting, or losing track of, what do you fear might happen?" Sometimes patients will intentionally suppress or conceal aspects of their thoughts and feelings, while at other times, resistances are unconscious and will come to patients' attention only through the therapist's activity.

Regardless of whether resistances are conscious or unconscious, analysis of resistance begins with pointing out that a defensive operation has been activated, followed by exploration of the motivation for defense. This will ultimately lead to uncovering and exploring the underlying conflictual motivations that are being defended against, enacted as an object relation in the transference. In essence, resistances are object relations, associated with a specific anxiety, that are activated in the treatment setting and enacted in the transference.

CLINICAL ILLUSTRATION OF ANALYSIS OF RESISTANCE

As an example of analysis of resistance, let us return to our 34-year-old professional woman discussed earlier in this chapter, who was stuck in a frustrating relationship with an unavailable man. The patient was describing a situation at work in which she had been selected to be the lead person on a project for an important account. The assignment came directly from the senior partner in her company, a highly influential and charismatic man in his mid-60s, who had a paternal yet slightly flirtatious relationship with the patient. The patient went on to say that she was sure she had been selected for this job because it was summer, and no one else wanted to take on a big project that might interfere with vacation. She was thinking that maybe she should cancel her vacation plans in advance in order to avoid any conflict. The patient confided in the therapist that she found herself feeling resentful, that her boss had no concern for her needs, and that she had been selected because of her difficulty in saying "No."

The therapist's initial internal reaction was to feel protective of the patient and concerned that she was allowing herself to be exploited by her powerful and much-admired boss. However, as he listened further, the therapist was struck by the patient's denial of the significance of the assignment in relation to her status in the firm and in her boss's eyes. The therapist asked for *clarification*, and, indeed, it turned out that the patient had been chosen for this important assignment over a number of her colleagues, many of them senior to her, though she had not really thought about this. As the therapist inquired further, it became quite evident that the assignment was a public statement on the part of her boss that he saw the patient as an important and valued member of the firm, more a reward than a sign of exploitation. The therapist was struck by the patient's apparent denial of all this in her initial telling of the story. At the same time, he made note of his own initial reaction of feeling sorry for and protective of the patient, rather than admiring of her success.

The therapist understood the patient's omission as a form of resistance. He commented on the omission to the patient, suggesting that it seemed she had some anxiety about being seen as successful. In response, the patient acknowledged that she understood what he was saying but that she had never really thought about the positive side of the assignment. She asked the therapist if he thought this was strange, and she added that she hoped the therapist didn't think she was trying to show off by telling him about the assignment. At this point, the therapist was able to make the interpretation that it appeared to make the patient anxious to acknowledge her successes, because it left her feeling that the therapist might see her as a show off.

In this vignette, the patient's resistance became apparent in the discrepancy between the way she initially presented the story and the more complex picture that emerged over time. (Notice that material emerged only because the therapist did not take what the patent said at face value, instead using common sense to pick up on aspects of her telling of the story that did not entirely make sense and asked for clarification.) The patient's resistance was also manifested in the therapist's countertransference; the therapist initially viewed the patient as vulnerable and potentially taken advantage of, rather than as triumphantly receiving recognition of her talents.

For this patient, omissions in the telling of the story functioned as a resistance to fully acknowledging, both to herself and to the therapist, an image of herself as competitive and successful. The anxiety motivating her resistance was that if she presented herself as someone interested in success and capable of achieving it, she would be seen as a show-off. From the perspective of *resistance to the transference*, the patient was resisting activation and enactment in the transference of the relationship pattern of a winning young woman who enjoys "showing her stuff" to an admiring older man. Instead, the patient enacted the defensive object relation of a vulnerable and easily exploited child in relation to a sympathetic and protective parent. This object relation protected the patient from the anxiety of being disapproved of, which she associated with her wishes to show off her successes.

In DPHP, analysis of resistance to free and open communication will always progress from defensive omissions (e.g., this patient omitted acknowledgment of her success), to object relations representing the motivation for defense (e.g., the patient feared that the therapist would disapprove of her as a show-off), and ultimately to the underlying impulsive object relations (e.g., the patient wished to triumphantly "show her stuff" to the therapist).

CHARACTER ANALYSIS

At this point, we would like to introduce another form of resistance frequently encountered in DPHP, which we will refer to as *character resistance*. In DPHP, the patient's defensive personality traits, or character defenses, are quickly enacted in the treatment, where they function as character resistances. Thus far, we have discussed resistances in terms of roadblocks or omissions in the content of the patient's verbal communications to the therapist. Resistances of this kind can be conceptualized as a form of "not seeing," in which conflictual mental contents are repressed, denied, or disavowed in order to avoid anxiety.

In contrast, character resistances do not involve omissions tied to repression, splitting, or denial. Instead, character resistances involve enactments tied to activation of the patient's character defenses in the treatment. In DPHP, the patient's character traits will take on meaning as they are enacted in the transference as a particular defensive object relation. Thus, instead of omitting mental contents in order to avoid anxiety, character resistances involve enacting a defensive object relation to block the possibility of anxiety emerging.

CHARACTER ANALYSIS AND ANALYSIS OF DEFENSE

In psychotherapy, character traits or character defenses manifest as a characteristic attitude or cluster of behaviors on the part of the patient that will be enacted in the treatment and in relation to the therapist to ward off anxiety. Because character defenses are ego syntonic, the patient typically will not be aware of enacting them as resistances in the treatment. Further, because whatever the patient is doing in the treatment is also what he does routinely in his daily life, even when the therapist points out the patient's attitude or behavior, the patient may lack curiosity about the therapist's observation, brushing if off with an attitude of "this is just how I am." Typically, it will take repeated efforts on the part of the therapist, bringing the patient's attention to his behavior or attitude, for the patient to begin to feel that there is something worth considering with regard to the meaning of his behavior.

CLINICAL ILLUSTRATION OF CHARACTER RESISTANCE

Let us return to the patient presented earlier in this chapter who had difficulty expressing anger at his partner. This patient always spoke in muted tones in his psychotherapy sessions. Initially, the therapist did not make much of this and simply asked the patient to repeat what he had said or to speak up a bit. However, when the patient's behavior persisted, the therapist began to take notice of his habit of speaking in such hushed tones. The therapist asked the patient about his behavior, and the patient responded that this was "just a habit."

When the therapist inquired further, the patient explained that all his friends had noticed his tendency to mumble and that people were always asking him to speak up. When the therapist continued to express curiosity about the patient's inaudible communications, the patient asked the therapist not to "make anything of it," and assured the therapist that he would try to speak louder. It was only over time that the patient became aware of the automatic and involuntary nature of his behavior, and of the fact that, even though he intended to speak up, he invariably did not. At this point, for the first time, the patient began to feel curious about his own behavior.

Curiosity on the part of the patient implies that he has developed some sort of understanding that what he is doing is "motivated" and meaningful rather than just "habit." This awareness on the part of the patient puts the therapist in a position to offer a tentative hypothesis about the anxiety the behavior is designed to ward off. For example, the therapist of the patient who spoke inaudibly suggested that perhaps the patient spoke so softly out of a fear that, if he were to speak loudly, he might seem "too aggressive." In essence, in the patient's unconscious mind, speaking softly obviated the possibility of being seen as aggressive.

CHARACTER RESISTANCES AND CLASSICAL RESISTANCES

The vignette described in the previous subsection illustrates the relationship between classical resistances and character resistances, on the one hand, and between "analysis of resistance" and "character analysis," on the other. Initially, we described a "classical resistance," in which there was a block in the patient's verbal communications, reflecting the activation of repression or disavowal in relation to the expression of hostility. Confronting this resistance involved pointing out and exploring an omission, which led to identification and exploration of the anxiety motivating defense, enacted as an object relation of a therapist who would withdraw from an angry or critical patient.

In contrast, the character resistance did not manifest as a block or as an absence, but rather as a behavior or attitude that warded off anxiety. As long as the patient spoke sotto voce, he experienced himself as someone incapable of communicating anger. Confrontation of this resistance involved the therapist's repeatedly pointing out to the patient that he was doing something worthy of his curiosity. Only after enactment of the character resistance became somewhat ego dystonic was there room for consideration of what was motivating the behavior, and it was only at this point that it became possible to identify the anxiety motivating the patient's behavior: that if he were to speak up, he would become aware of his fear of seeming aggressive in the eyes of the therapist. The difference between the two forms of resistance is that, whereas the omission simply "deleted" awareness of the patient's anxiety about feeling angry or critical, the character resistance functioned to reassure the patient that there was no need for anxiety, by, in his mind, negating the possibility of being seen as aggressive.

The general approach to working with character resistances is, first, to bring them to the patient's attention, highlighting the unrealistic or unexpected nature of the patient's attitude or behavior. This process, which may take time and repeated confrontation on the part of the therapist, will make character defenses more visible, or less ego syntonic, to the patient. Once the patient becomes aware of and curious about his behavior, the next step is to explore the anxieties motivating the character resistance. At this point, the approach to character resistance and resistance to free association will converge, as attention is paid to the anxieties motivating the patient's defensive behavior.

INTERPRETATION AND CONTAINMENT

In our discussion of countertransference, we considered the process of containment from the perspective of the therapist's capacity to contain the affects and object relations activated in him by the patient's verbal and nonverbal communications. Here, containment of the countertransference provides the therapist with information about the object relations being enacted in the treatment, while preventing countertransference acting out. From this vantage point, containment is a process that goes on in the mind of the therapist and that functions as a preliminary step toward interpretation.

However, there is another perspective on containment. In this view, containment is viewed as an interpersonal interaction that takes place between patient and therapist and that, in and of itself, carries therapeutic potential (Bion 1959, 1962a, 1962b; Britton 1998; Ogden 1982; Steiner 1994). Before completing our discussion of the techniques of DPHP, we would like to comment on this second view of the role of containment in psychotherapy.

CONTAINMENT, TRIANGULATION, AND INTEGRATION

As we have described, containment begins when the patient induces affects and activates object relations in the therapist that in some way mirror or complement his own. The therapist contains his reactions to the patient by reflecting upon them and, in so doing, avoids responding either by reflexively mirroring back the patient's affective state or by complementing it—for example, by responding to the patient's hostility with hostility on the one hand or with fear on the other. Thus, containment entails two processes. First, the therapist must be able to accurately "read" the patient's affective state. This process reflects the therapist's openness to the patient, expressed in the therapist's capacity to be emotionally receptive, allowing the object relations enacted in the treatment to affect him internally. Second, the therapist must also in some way observe what is being enacted in the transference–countertransference, therein subtly creating a distance between himself and the immediate situation.

The therapist's capacity to do both of these tasks—to both accurately perceive and emotionally experience the internal object relations enacted in the treatment on the one hand, and to reflect upon his internal experience on the other—will ensure that while the therapist's emotional experience will correspond with that of the patient, at the same time, it will not be exactly congruent with that of the patient. As a result of the process of containment, the therapist responds, but does not simply respond "in kind," to the patient's projections; the therapist adds a new perspective (Kernberg 2004b).

We think of this two-part process as a form of "triangulation" within the mind of the therapist, in which, on the one hand, the therapist identifies with the patient's self or object representations, and, on the other, uses his own internal capacity for self-observation to reflect upon his experience. This capacity on the part of the therapist—to accurately read and to empathize with, while at the same time maintaining a sense of differentiation from, the patient—is implicitly communicated to the patient. Fonagy and Target (2003) have described this aspect of containment in terms of the therapist's "marking" the patient's affective state, communicating that he appreciates the patient's emotional situation and is affected by it but does not entirely share the patient's experience and is not overwhelmed by it. These authors have linked this process to the development of the capacity, both developmentally in the young child and clinically in the adult patient, to reflect upon affective experience.

We have been describing the capacity of the containing therapist to reflect back to the patient an accurate recognition of the patient's emotional state, and also an implicit perspective on that experience. The therapist's capacity to, in this way, serve a containing function for the patient is of particular importance in settings where the patient's affect state is especially intense and the associated object relations are especially threatening. For example, if the patient is intensely angry or frightened, or if he is feeling sexually stimulated in the session, the therapist's capacity to contain and metabolize the patient's affective experience becomes extremely important. In his containing function, the therapist creates in his own mind a more highly integrated version of the patient's experience, helping the patient to better tolerate and modulate potentially overwhelming affect states (Bion 1959, 1962a, 1962b).

"THERAPIST-CENTERED INTERPRETATION" AND CONTAINMENT

When affect activation is high, thinking may become more concrete, and it may be difficult for a patient to take in the meaning of the therapist's words. For example, if a patient is feeling enraged, and the therapist makes an accurate interpretation about the patient's hostility or about the patient's fears in relation to his own hostility, the patient may feel attacked by the therapist. Similarly, if the therapist interprets the patient's anxieties about having sexual feelings, the patient may feel that the therapist is being overtly seductive, regardless of the actual content of what the therapist is saying. In essence, in situations of this kind, the object relations activated in the treatment are experienced as if they are actually being played out interpersonally with the therapist.

While situations of this kind are far more commonly encountered in the treatments of patients with severe personality disorders, they can also be seen in patients with higher level personality pathology. In DPHP, the therapist's capacity to contain the object relations enacted in the transference can help the patient convert an intense and threatening affective experience that he has limited capacity to reflect upon into a better modulated affective experience that leaves greater room for self-reflection.

At times when highly affectively charged object relations are activated in the treatment, it is often best for the therapist to begin by simply putting the patient's experience into words. For example, the therapist might say "You are feeling enraged with your brother." Similarly, when highly charged object relations are enacted in relation to the therapist, it is often best to make a "therapist-centered interpretation" (Steiner 1994)—one in which the therapist simply comments on the patient's experience of the therapist. For example, the therapist may say, "You feel that I am attacking you," or "When I comment on sexual feelings in the session, it confuses you and leaves you feeling that I am trying to seduce you." Therapist-centered interpretations serve a containing function, helping the patient to tolerate extremely painful affective experiences, by accurately registering what the patient is feeling and putting it into words; the therapist's words present the patient with a better integrated version of highly affectively charged and relatively poorly integrated internal experiences that the patient has not been able to tolerate. At the same time, implicit in a therapist-centered interpretation is demonstration that the therapist can tolerate what the patient cannot tolerate experiencing and that, in contrast to the patient, the therapist is not swept away in the transference–countertransference and is able to reflect on what is happening between them.

At other times of high-affect intensity, the therapist may choose not to offer an interpretation. Here, the therapist's containing function will be communicated to the patient nonverbally through his tone of voice and facial expression. In this situation, the therapist's capacity to allow himself to be affected by the patient's emotional state without reflexively mirroring back to the patient affects of similar intensity and without acting out in the countertransference may help the patient better tolerate his own affects.

CONTAINMENT AS A THERAPEUTIC PROCESS

In DPHP, both interpretations and non-interpretive forms of containment implicitly communicate that the therapist can tolerate what the patient is experiencing and projecting without being overly threatened or becoming overwhelmed or lost in the experience. In fact, this stance replicates what the therapist hopes to help the patient accomplish, that is, to become able to tolerate awareness of threatening and highly affectively charged object relations while maintaining the capacity to reflect upon them. This capacity will enable the patient to explore his internal experience when highly conflictual object relations are activated and enacted in the treatment. Ultimately, the capacity to contain—to tolerate awareness of conflictual object relations and highly charged affect states and then to reflect upon them without necessarily automatically acting upon them or trying to make them disappear—corresponds to the overall goal of DPHP, that of integrating conflictual experiences of self and other into the dominant sense of self.

The perspective on containment that we have presented suggests that whenever a therapist makes a meaningful interpretation to a patient who is affectively involved, the therapist is serving as a "container," as well as an "interpreter" of the patient's mental experience. From this perspective, interpretations both explain and contain, and explaining functions as a form of containment. The explanatory aspects of interpretation, communicated in the meaning of the therapist's words, function to contain intense affect states and threatening object relations by putting feelings into words and providing additional perspective on the patient's mental experience.

We believe that in DPHP, the explanatory and containing functions of interpretation work together to promote the kind of integration of conflictual object relations that is the goal of the treatment. In our theory of technique, we focus explicitly on the exploration and interpretation of affectively charged, conflictual object relations, in order to promote integration. However, the containing function of the psychotherapeutic relationship is implicit in the technique of DPHP. Along with interpretation, the therapist's neutral stance and his listening, concern, restraint, and "marking," all serve a containing function, helping the patient to tolerate awareness of and better integrate highly threatening and affectively charged, conflictual object relations. In the end, we hope to enhance the patient's capacity to contain his own conflictual object relations—in essence, fulfilling the function previously carried out by the "containing therapist."

SUGGESTED READINGS

Kernberg OF: Convergences and divergences in contemporary psychoanalytic technique, in Contemporary Controversies in Psychoanalytic Theory, Techniques, and Their Applications. New Haven, CT, Yale University Press, 2004, pp 267–284

LaFarge L: Interpretation and containment. Int J Psychoanalysis 81:67–84, 2000

Levy ST, Inderbitzin LB: Neutrality, interpretation and therapeutic intent. J Am Psychoanal Assn 40:989–1011, 1992

Reich A: Character Analysis. New York, Noonday Press, 1949

Samberg E, Marcus E: Process, resistance, and interpretation, in The American Psychiatric Publishing Textbook of Psychoanalysis. Edited by Person ES, Cooper AM, Gabbard GO. Washington, DC, American Psychiatric Publishing, 2005, pp 229–240

Schafer R: Resisting and empathizing, in The Analytic Attitude. New York, Basic Books, 1983, pp 66–81

Schafer R: The analysis of resistance, in The Analytic Attitude. New York, Basic Books, 1983, pp 162–182

Steiner J: Patient-centered and analyst-centered interpretations. Psychoanalytic Inquiry 14:406–422, 1994

8

THE TACTICS OF DPHP

So far, we have described the overall strategy the therapist uses in dynamic psychotherapy for higher level personality pathology (DPHP) to promote integration of conflictual object relations, with the goal of reducing personality rigidity in specified areas of functioning, and the treatment setting within which these strategies are implemented. We have also described the specific techniques employed by the therapist, moment to moment, to achieve this aim. We now address the tactics of DPHP.

Conceptually, tactics form the link between the strategies of the treatment as a whole and the moment-to-moment interventions made by the therapist. Practically, these tactics guide the therapist in each session as he decides how to implement the techniques, described in the previous chapter, in the service of meeting the central objectives of the treatment. Tactics guide decision making with regard to where, when, and how to intervene (Table 8–1).

TACTIC 1: WHERE TO INTERVENE— IDENTIFYING A PRIORITY THEME

In DPHP, each session will have one or two issues that, if one were to stand back and listen to the session, would emerge as organizing themes. We refer to this material as the *priority theme* or *central issue* in the session. Some of the patient's communications will present the central issue and other material will defend against it, but once the therapist has determined the priority theme for the session, the material will fall into place conceptually. The central issue or priority theme is similar to Bion's (1967b) concept of the *selected fact*.

In DPHP, some issues are introduced by the things the patient says, and others through nonverbal communication. There are issues the patient is aware of bringing into the session, and there are also issues that the patient is defending against acknowledging. The first tactic of the DPHP therapist is to select a priority theme for the session and to identify the dominant object relations embedded in that theme. The priority theme will correspond to the dominant conflicts and conflictual object relations currently being enacted or defended against in the session. As a result, when selecting a priority theme we look for indications of the activation of unconscious conflict.

To choose a priority theme for the immediate session and moment, the therapist first considers whether the patient is communicating openly and freely. If he is, the therapist next considers which material is affectively dominant in the patient's verbal and nonverbal communications. If the priority theme remains unclear, the therapist can ask himself what are the predominant object relations being enacted in the transference, followed by what is being stimulated in the countertransference.

RESISTANCE TO FREE AND OPEN COMMUNICATION

When trying to determine a priority theme, the therapist should always begin by asking himself whether anything appears to be interfering with the patient's communicating openly and freely with the therapist. Does the patient appear to be holding back information? Is he having difficulty speaking freely? If the answer to either of these questions is yes, the therapist can infer that the conflicts associated with the patient's difficulty in communicating freely are the central issue in the session at that moment. This is to say that, when the patient is not communicating openly, his behavior is typically motivated by concerns reflecting the activation of conflictual object relations. In this setting, exploring the patient's difficulty being open with the therapist becomes the priority theme in the session.

AFFECTIVE DOMINANCE

If the patient is speaking freely, the therapist next turns his attention to the patient's verbal and nonverbal communications to identify a priority theme. When determining which material to pursue, the therapist is guided by the

---

TABLE 8–1. Tactics of dynamic psychotherapy for higher level personality pathology (DPHP)

Tactic 1	Identifying a "priority theme": where to intervene
Tactic 2	Defining the conflict
Tactic 3	Analyzing the dominant conflict systematically, from defense to conflictual motivation
Tactic 4	Analyzing the relationship between the dominant conflict and the treatment goals

---

principle of affective dominance, also referred to as the *economic principle of interpretation* (Fenichel 1941). The principle of affective dominance directs the therapist to intervene in relation to the material in which the patient has invested the most affect. The rationale for this approach is that the activation of conflictual mental contents stimulates affects as well as defenses against these affects. As a result, we look for affective investment to signal the activation of conflictual object relations.

It is important to understand that affective dominance reflects affective or emotional *investment* in the material in question and that this will not always be accompanied by an overt display of emotion. In fact, sometimes affective dominance is reflected in the patient's failure to express expectable emotion, indicating that the activation of conflictual object relations is stimulating defensive operations and that affect is being suppressed, repressed, or dissociated. For example, a patient may describe an objectively frightening experience in a calm, detached manner. At other times, affective dominance is reflected in the content of the patient's communications, for example, in the repetitive description of particular object relations or in his nonverbal communications.

When significant affect accompanies apparently thoughtful discussion of a particular issue, it suggests that the material being considered is affectively dominant in the session. For example, if a patient is remembering packing up his daughter's belongings to take her to college, and in sharing these memories with the therapist the patient becomes tearful, we can infer that whatever conflicts are expressed in his tearful remembrance of his daughter's leaving home are likely affectively dominant at the moment.

Conversely, when affect is strikingly absent from a patient's discussion of a particular topic, it also typically signifies affective dominance. Here, the absence of emotion indicates that the activation of conflictual object relations is stimulating defensive operations. For example, if a patient is speaking apparently freely and openly about the marital problems that brought him to treatment, but he is doing so in a manner that seems distanced from the material and is emotionally flat, we can infer that conflicts activated in discussing his marital problems are highly invested with affect. Similarly, if the patient's affect is discordant with material he is discussing, this is also suggestive of affective dominance. In this case, the therapist should ask the patient to clarify the apparent incongruity. For example, the therapist might say something along the lines of, "You are talking about painful problems in your marriage, problems that brought you to treatment, yet you don't seem concerned. In fact, your manner is almost cheerful. What are your thoughts about this?"

Sometimes affective dominance will be signaled less by the presence or absence of affect expression and more by the content of the patient's communications. Here, we may see the repetitive description of one or two themes or constellations of object relations, in different forms and contexts, through the course of the session. Sometimes one of the object relations will be enacted in the transference as well.

When looking to the contents of the patient's communications for affective dominance, the therapist should keep in mind that in DPHP the activation of unconscious conflict is not always expressed exclusively or even predominantly through verbal communication. It is not uncommon for defensively activated object relations to be communicated through subtle behavioral gestures or to be expressed and enacted in the quality of interaction between patient and therapist. For example, it might be more important for the therapist to focus on the fact that the patient is failing to make eye contact or seems overly ingratiating than on the content of what the patient is saying. In fact, when the patient's behavior is incongruent with his words and the affective dominance is unclear, behavior is probably more important than content and should be explored first.

ADDITIONAL APPROACHES TO SELECTING A PRIORITY THEME

Sometimes it will be difficult to determine affective dominance. When this is the case, we suggest that the therapist first carefully reconsider whether the patient is communicating openly and freely or holding back or having difficulty. If there are no apparent blocks to open communication, we suggest the therapist next consider what might be going on in the *transference*, as reflected in the patient's remarks and behavior. If things still remain unclear, it can be helpful to carefully consider the *countertransference* because it may provide a guide to defense, anxiety, and hidden affect. If no significant theme has yet emerged, the therapist should continue to listen and evaluate the ongoing flow of material, waiting until an affectively dominant theme presents itself.

It is not unusual for the therapist to find it difficult to establish affectively dominant themes at particular junctures in the treatment. However, if this happens repeatedly or over an extended period of time, it may reflect conscious suppression of material on the part of the patient. If this is the case, the patient's suppression is the priority theme in the session. In this situation, the therapist should explore the patient's defensive operations, defining the conflicts and anxieties underlying the patient's difficulty with regard to openly communicating in sessions.

During periods when a priority theme cannot be identified and the therapist is having difficulty organizing the material in a meaningful way, it can be tempting to pick a theme arbitrarily. We strongly recommend against doing this. The therapist's directing the session in this way is likely to lead only to intellectualized exploration of the material. If the therapist is patient and does not intrude or direct the session, limiting interventions only to analysis of resistance, the dominant theme will ultimately come into focus.

In sum, with regard to choosing a priority theme, a combined analysis of the patient's communications about his thoughts and feelings, the therapist's observations of what the patient says and does, and examination of the countertransference should lead to a determination of the most important issue at the moment.

TACTIC 2: DEFINING THE CONFLICT

Having identified the priority theme, the therapist wants to define the conflict that this issue represents. This is accomplished by identifying the object relations that represent the priority issue and then considering their defensive and expressive functions. As the therapist receives the patient's verbal and nonverbal communications, the therapist constructs in his own mind descriptions of the internal object relations representing the patient's communications around the priority theme. The experienced DPHP therapist does this automatically, hearing the patient's communications in terms of relationship patterns. The less experienced therapist can make a conscious effort to transform verbal and nonverbal communications into patterned object relations.

IDENTIFYING THE DEFENSE

Once the therapist has defined the array of object relations associated with the priority theme, he now wants to consider how they fit together with regard to conflict and defense. As the therapist considers these object relations, the first question he asks himself is "Where is the defense?" As we have discussed, relationship patterns serving defensive purposes will be conscious, close to the surface of the patient's psychological experience, and relatively acceptable to the patient. The therapist can make use of this to identify relationship patterns defensively activated in the session by considering the questions "What are the dominant images of self and of others that the patient is describing?" and "How is the patient consciously experiencing himself in the session?"

IDENTIFYING THE ANXIETY MOTIVATING DEFENSE AND THE UNDERLYING CONFLICTUAL MOTIVATION

Having defined an array of object relations associated with the priority theme of the session and having located the defensive object relations among them, the therapist next constructs hypotheses about the conflict being defended against. Defining a conflict entails identifying the defense; the anxiety motivating the defense—that is, the psychological dangers associated with expression of conflictual motivations or their emergence into consciousness; and the underlying conflictual motivation, expressed as a highly motivated, wished-for, feared, or needed relationship. All will be embedded in the object relations associated with the conflict.

Moving from surface to depth, after identifying the defensive object relations, the therapist considers the anxiety motivating the defense. The *anxiety motivating defense* refers to the affects and concerns that the patient hopes to avoid by enacting defensive relationship patterns. These anxieties will generally be relatively accessible to consciousness; if they are not conscious at the moment, they will have been so in the past and will feel familiar to the patient when identified. To identify the anxiety motivating a defense, the therapist can ask himself, "What feelings and concerns is the patient avoiding by experiencing himself or an object as he has constructed them in the defensive object relation?" "What would the patient feel if he were to view himself or the object differently in this situation?" and "What would he feel if the roles were reversed?"

Having identified the anxiety that is motivating defense, the therapist can move on to consider the conflictual motivation or relationship pattern that underlies the dominant conflict. The conflictual motivation typically will be the aspect of any given conflict that is least accessible to the patient. Here, the therapist considers, "What is it within himself that the patient is most afraid of at this moment?" and "What is the patient attempting to bury as a result of his defensive operations?" Each of the questions the therapist asks himself in the process of defining a conflict can be answered by describing an object relation. In his efforts to define the conflict, the therapist will call upon his dynamic and structural understanding of the patient's inner life, along with his countertransference.

WHY NOW?

When defining the conflict presently enacted or defended against in the treatment, the therapist should always be asking himself, "Why is this conflict being activated now?" In considering this question, the therapist should keep in mind recent events in the patient's life and in his treatment. Life events will activate conflicts and defenses that will be enacted in the treatment. At the same time, conflicts and defenses activated by the treatment can precipitate events in the patient's daily life. As a result, keeping the realities of the patient's life situation in mind will provide a context for the therapist as he tries to put together the data assembled from affective, dynamic, and structural considerations.

Similarly, keeping in mind the material that was discussed in the previous session or two will also help guide the therapist as he approaches the material the patient presents in a given session. In DPHP, there is a process from session to session that tends to become more autonomous and less driven by day-to-day events as the treatment progresses. In this process, the therapy takes on something of a life of its own, and the therapist can often best understand the conflicts and defenses enacted in a given session as reactions to or continuation of material explored in the previous sessions. In the same way that life events stimulate conflict and defense, so do recent events in the treatment. It is helpful for the therapist to keep in mind that changes in the frame—for example, interruptions for vacations or even a single missed appointment or a change of meeting time—can sometimes stimulate powerful reactions.

CLINICAL ILLUSTRATION OF SELECTING A PRIORITY THEME AND IDENTIFYING THE CONFLICT

Let's return to the female patient discussed in the section on countertransference in Chapter 6 ("The Techniques of DPHP, Part 1: Listening to the Patient"). The patient is 45 years old, professionally successful, and single. She has been in treatment for 6 months. She has maintained a positive, somewhat idealized relationship with the therapist. The patient tends to feel down if she misses a therapy session. The therapist has pointed this out, but the patient does not like to believe that the schedule of her sessions has anything to do with the fluctuations in her mood. In fact, she rarely thinks about the therapist or about the treatment between sessions.

In the session we described, the patient had been talking excitedly about the details of a wonderful weekend with her new boyfriend. The patient's tone was excited, and she was laughing, apparently having great fun sharing all this with the therapist, as though speaking with a close friend or comrade who experienced equally exciting weekends. Initially, the therapist was swept up in the patient's manic mood, feeling excited herself and wanting to laugh along with the patient. However, as the therapist continued to listen, she started to feel diminished and demoralized. She found herself thinking about how the patient had things the therapist herself would never have and that her own life seemed colorless and boring in comparison.

The therapist felt that the priority issue in the session was the contrast between the mutual idealization and excitement of the early part of the session and the growing feeling of demoralization that then replaced these in the countertransference. This struck the therapist as analogous to the contrast between how the patient felt in the session and how she felt when she missed a session. The therapist proceeded, in her own mind, to *describe the object relations* she had identified in the patient's communications. First, there was the excited couple enacted in the session. There was the dependent patient who needed her nurturing therapist to sustain her mood. There was the patient who did not want to acknowledge feeling dependent and did not think about her therapist between sessions. Finally, there was the object relation experienced in the countertransference—that of someone who "had it all" while someone else felt inferior and excluded. In this last relationship pattern, hostility was denied by both parties.

Next, the therapist asked herself, "Where is the defense?" She identified the object relation of the excited couple and the atmosphere of contagious excitement that characterized much of the session as reflecting activation of the patient's "manic" defenses. The therapist reflected on the relationship enacted, of two successful and triumphant insiders swept away by the excitement of sharing successes that they both enjoyed. The therapist noted that, in this object relation, self and object were more alike than different, like two girlfriends sharing their exploits. There was no sense of a doctor–patient relationship or a dependent relationship of any kind. The patient consciously experienced this object relation, enacted with the therapist.

Consideration of the patient's manic defenses led the therapist to the *anxiety motivating the patient's defensive operations.* It was clear that the patient was doing what she could to avoid acknowledging feelings of dependency. The therapist considered, "What would the patient feel if she were to acknowledge feeling dependent on me?" The therapist made a link to her experience in the countertransference of feeling excluded and inferior. The therapist hypothesized that the patient's defensive stance was motivated by anxiety and painful feelings associated with being in a dependent position, which, for the patient, was experienced in terms of needing someone who had it all and who did not need her in return, and risking feeling inferior and unwanted. These anxieties were quite close to the surface, and the therapist anticipated that as soon as the patient calmed down and was less well protected by her defenses, this painful object relation would become accessible.

The therapist then considered the underlying motivation and why it was conflictual. The patient seemed to be avoiding experiencing herself in a relationship in which she was vulnerable and dependent upon a figure from whom she wanted love and care at the risk of pain and humiliation. On the basis of previous knowledge that she had of the patient and her history, the therapist inferred that more deeply buried were representations of dependent relationships colored by envy and sadism.

At this point, the therapist considered, "Why now?" She thought of the patient's growing attachment to her new boyfriend. She also thought of her own upcoming summer vacation, which would interrupt the treatment for several weeks. Apparently, both were stimulating anxieties in the patient about feeling left behind, dependent, and excluded.

By this point, the therapist felt quite able to define the conflict currently active in the treatment. Clearly, the patient's increasing investment in the relationship with the boyfriend and in her treatment, in conjunction with anticipation of the therapist's leaving on vacation, had intensified conflicts around dependency. Closest to the surface and at times conscious were the anxieties motivating the patient's defensive operations. We refer here to the patient's feelings of being left behind, excluded, and inferior. These concerns were defended against using manic defenses that denied exclusion, dependency, or difference between patient and therapist. Less accessible to the patient were more aggressive and envious object relations associated with dependent object relations.

At this point, the therapist thought about how best to intervene.

TACTIC 3: SYSTEMATIC ANALYSIS OF THE DOMINANT CONFLICT

Systematic analysis of unconscious conflict is the cornerstone of DPHP, and virtually everything in this handbook deals with how to carry out this tactic. Here we describe general principles that guide the therapist's approach.

As we have discussed, DPHP is embedded in a model of the mind in which object relations are activated and enacted according to the defensive needs of the patient. Enactment of defensive object relations supports repression of underlying object relations. Defensive object relations are generally relatively realistic, nonthreatening, and ego syntonic. In contrast, object relations more directly tied to underlying wishes, needs, and fears are generally less realistic, more threatening, and more highly affectively charged.

The overall approach in DPHP is to systematically analyze the object relations enacted in the treatment, beginning with those activated in the service of defense. In this process, we uncover representations of self and other that have been repressed and/or dissociated from the patient's conscious self experience. As the defensive functions of a particular internal object relation are elaborated and interpreted, the underlying conflict will come into focus.

GUIDING PRINCIPLES OF CONFLICT ANALYSIS— FROM SURFACE TO DEPTH

In DPHP, we always begin our interventions with the material closest to consciousness and move toward material that is less accessible. This principle is referred to as the *dynamic principle of interpretation* (Fenichel 1941). This principle states that when analyzing a conflict, one should think in terms of which elements are defensive and which are defended against and intervene first at the level of material that is defensive. This approach is often described in terms of moving, metaphorically, *from surface to depth*. This is because, by definition, defensive internal object relations are closest to consciousness and relatively acceptable to the patient, whereas object relations that are defended against are more highly conflictual and more difficult to consciously tolerate. When intervening, we begin at the surface, exploring the relatively acceptable representations being enacted, and we move, in the session as well as through the course of the treatment, toward exploration of more deeply repressed and unacceptable aspects of psychological experience.

GUIDING PRINCIPLES OF CONFLICT ANALYSIS— DISSOCIATION BEFORE REPRESSION

Many patients with higher level personality pathology present with defensive relationship patterns that clearly reflect the use of splitting-based defenses. In this setting, it is generally best to confront and explore dissociation and denial before analyzing defensive operations that are based on repression. This is consistent with our overall approach of beginning with those object relations that are closest to consciousness. As the dissociation of conflicting motivations is confronted and explored, the conflicts and associated anxieties avoided by dissociation will emerge.

As an example of the approach we are recommending, consider the businesswoman who presents complaining of an inability to assert herself with her live-in boyfriend. This patient owns and runs a large and successful business, where she has many people reporting to her and is a forceful leader who does not shy away from confrontation. In her social life, she has always been equally assertive, frequently assuming a leadership role among her friends. However, for the first time, she is in love. What she has discovered—and what brings her to treatment—is that when she is home alone with her boyfriend, she finds herself timid in an unfamiliar way and fearful of asserting herself in even the most neutral and seemingly reasonable fashion.

In this patient's treatment, we would begin by confronting her use of dissociation. This would entail describing the object relations associated with the patient's familiar self experience and pointing out how starkly this sense of herself in relation to others contrasts with how she feels and behaves with her boyfriend. We might, in addition, point out the degree to which she denies how dramatically differently she behaves when home alone with her boyfriend. After defining and exploring the object relations associated with these two dissociated aspects of the patient's experience, we would suggest to her that the dissociation of her tender self from her usual businesswoman self must protect her from anxiety; it is as though she is afraid to introduce her familiar, assertive, and powerful self into the interactions with her boyfriend.

As the therapist consistently confronts dissociation and denial and helps the patient explore the functions served by compartmentalizing her internal experience in this way, the patient's defenses will become less ego syntonic and at the same time less effective. This will leave room to begin exploration of underlying anxieties that have been avoided by dissociation—in this case, the patient's concerns about being powerful in the setting of dependent relations and, ultimately, her anxiety about being in a dependent position herself.

In the absence of evident use of dissociative defenses, we turn to analysis of repression-based defenses. When analyzing dissociative defenses, we looked for the polarization of conflictual motivations *between* conflicting object relations along with denial of the significance of conscious object relations that are conflictual. In contrast, when analyzing repression-based defenses, it can be helpful to consider the degree to which conflicting motivations are polarized *within* the defensive object relations enacted in the treatment. This combination reflects the use of neurotic projection. In this setting, we can observe a polarized quality to the patient's conscious experience of himself in interaction with others. We may see a defensive object relation, for example, in which the object is very powerful and the self dependent and powerless, or the object very sexual and the self indifferent and free of sexual interest. Meanwhile, the patient has no awareness of feeling powerful or of having sexual feelings.

Guided once again by the principle of starting from material that is conscious, in this situation we typically begin our intervention by addressing the polarized quality of the representations coloring the patient's subjective experience. The therapist first helps the patient characterize the self and object representations being enacted, along with the different sets of motivations associated with each role. Next the therapist points out to the patient how one representation or internal object relation is very powerful, or very sexual, while the other representation is not at all so but is instead associated with an entirely different set of motivations.

Having described the relevant object relations, focusing on the polarized quality of the representations and the segregation of motivations, the therapist will introduce the idea that the patient's repetitive experience of himself in a particular relationship pattern is a construction rather than a reasonable view of external reality. The patient's appreciation that he is actively organizing his experience in a particular, albeit painful or maladaptive, fashion paves the way for exploration of the defensive functions served by repetitive enactment of these object relations. The final step is to define the underlying conflict associated with the defensive operations that have been identified.

If there is no apparent use of either dissociation or projection in the defensive object relations being enacted in the session, we turn to the analysis of repression proper. Here, we consider the ways in which the relationship patterns that the patient is enacting function to support repression of other object relations that are more conflictual. As always, we begin by characterizing the representations and motivations associated with defensive object relations and, in the process, we bring to the patient's attention how he repetitively and rigidly constructs his experience to enact these particular relationship patterns. The patient's gradual recognition that he is actively organizing his experience in a particular fashion paves the way to exploration of the defensive functions served by the repetitive enactment of these object relations. Over time, in conjunction with analysis of resistance, this will open the door to an exploration of the underlying, more highly conflictual object relations that have been repressed by virtue of the defensive object relations that are being enacted.

CLINICAL ILLUSTRATION OF SYSTEMATIC ANALYSIS OF THE DOMINANT CONFLICT

Let us consider the 40-year-old married male professional with conflicts around anger and authority. The patient presented with complaints of feeling inadequate with regard to power and money, especially relative to his friends' accomplishments. In the initial consultation, it became clear that the patient was reasonably successful within his profession but was inhibited in pursuing opportunities that would be more lucrative or would put him in a more influential position.

In one session, the patient presented a series of situations from the previous week in which he had been unable to assert himself or to pursue opportunities that would foster his professional advancement. Instead, he had allowed himself to be taken advantage of, and he felt like a loser. The therapist identified the patient's inhibitions, his submissiveness, and the feeling of being a loser as the priority issue; the patient enacted an object relation of a loser who perpetually submitted to a superior and powerful authority figure. This was the object relation closest to the surface and functioned as a character defense.

The therapist responded to the patient's description of himself by commenting, "It is as if you have a particular image of yourself interacting with someone you see as powerful, and you replay this scenario over and over again. You view yourself as a loser, someone who is inferior and weak. Then you rationalize that on this basis that you must be submissive, that there is no way you can even consider asserting yourself. You tell yourself you would only humiliate yourself by trying."

The patient interrupted the therapist, saying, "Hearing you say that only makes me feel worse, like you're telling me I'm a loser! And the fact that I see a therapist twice a week makes me even *more* of a loser."

At this point, the therapist had to decide whether to confront the enactment in the transference or, instead, to identify for the patient the defensive functions served by the relationship pattern of an inferior "loser" in relation to someone more powerful. The therapist knew that if he pointed out to the patient that the patient was experiencing exactly the situation with the therapist that the therapist was describing, then the patient would only feel criticized and humiliated. As a result, the therapist decided to wait to make this intervention, with the expectation that, down the road, the patient would be more open to it.

Instead, the therapist told the patient, "In my view, you feel like a loser because this is how you need to see it. You need to feel that I see you as a loser and that your efforts to better or advance yourself only betray weakness and will lead to humiliation. I think you need to see things this way because, painful as it is, it protects you; it keeps you safe."

The patient responded by telling the therapist that now he felt as though the therapist were only trying to make him feel better—as though the therapist were saying, "You're not really a loser—you just think you're a loser."

The therapist responded, "This is exactly my point. It's as though you will do anything and everything to hang onto the image of yourself as a loser." The patient seemed more reflective and then asked why the therapist thought he found it safe to feel like a loser when it made him so miserable. The therapist replied, "That's a very good question. What I notice is how polarized your image is, the image of yourself in relation to someone whom you see as in a position of power or authority. One person is absolutely powerful and in charge; the other absolutely powerless and submissive, a loser. It is as if you are afraid to see yourself as having even a drop of assertiveness, let alone power, or to see yourself as anything but a loser—as if that would be dangerous or would frighten you."

The patient considered how he felt when he had met with his boss earlier that day: intimidated as always, even though he really did not think much of this man. The patient had promised himself that he would use the meeting to bring up the topic of a long-promised promotion. Yet, once again, the patient had let his boss give him the runaround. His boss had turned the conversation to how tight the budget was, and the patient felt inhibited about returning to his agenda. The patient imagined that, if he pushed it, he would appear "self-important and greedy."

The therapist responded to the patient's comment by pointing out that it seemed one reason the patient tended to see himself as powerless, submissive, and a loser was that he feared that if he asserted himself, he would appear self-important and greedy. The therapist added that "self-important and greedy" was the same description that the patient often used in regard to his boss. It was as though, in the patient's mind, whoever was the boss or had the power became, in the patient's words, "a selfish, greedy asshole." The only alternative was to feel powerless. The patient acknowledged that this was a familiar, conscious concern. It probably was not realistic, but it was something he always worried about. It was as though he thought he would "become" his mother.

That night, the patient had a nightmare of watching a man verbally attack a woman. The man appeared to be on the brink of physical violence. Maybe he could kill her! The patient was frightened for himself and at the same time felt guilty that he was not able to protect the woman. He tried to reach the woman, but a door was locked. Yet maybe he was not trying hard enough because he was afraid. Shouldn't he call "911"?

The therapist noted to himself that, embedded in the manifest content of the dream, there was an object relation underlying the selfish greedy boss and the powerless loser. The object relation represented in the dream, and otherwise outside the patient's awareness, more closely reflected the patient's sadism and his fears of losing control of it than did the material previously discussed in the treatment. In the relationship pattern portrayed by the dream, the patient feared he or his object would become overtly sadistic and aggressive and, in fact, dangerous. The therapist appreciated that, even though the conflict was directly represented in the dream, the sadistic object relation was still otherwise quite far from the patient's awareness. (The closest manifestation in the session was the patient's expectation that the therapist would humiliate him.)

After listening to the patient's associations, the therapist made an interpretation with regard to the patient's underlying anxieties about his sadism: "I suspect that this dream is a response to our session yesterday and our discussion about your becoming anxious when you see yourself as powerful. Although these concerns are largely out of your awareness, your dream suggests that you are fearful of having power, at least in part, because in your mind, power leads to a frightening loss of control. It is as if you have these impulses inside you that have to be kept under wraps. You feel that if these impulses are ever unleashed, you will be unable to protect other people from your rage and potential violence."

The therapist made this interpretation with the expectation that it would have little impact, because the material was not currently active beyond its representation in the dream. He also anticipated, however, that the patient's concerns about his sadism and about being treated sadistically would emerge down the road in a more affectively meaningful way and that he would then be able to refer back to the dream and the interpretation made at that time.

This vignette illustrates the approach to confronting and interpreting projection and the defensive segregation of conflicting motivations embedded in a single object relation. The patient had separated power from dependency and in so doing had made himself totally powerless. The therapist began by pointing out to the patient that he attributed all the power in the relationship to the other person, leaving himself entirely powerless, dependent, and submissive. The therapist then raised the defensive nature of this object relation. Next, he identified the anxiety motivating the defense: the fear that if the patient were to be powerful, he would also become self-important and greedy. The next step would be to explore the underlying impulse and the dangers associated with its expression, as represented in the dream material but otherwise unconscious.

For the moment, the therapist anticipated that as he continued to confront and interpret the dissociation in the powerful-submissive object relation and also looked for opportunities to point out how this object relation was enacted in the transference, the powerful representation and the dependent representation would become less starkly separated. In this setting, the patient would gradually be able to see himself as other than powerless. This shift would open up the patient to becoming more aware of (i.e., more anxious about) the underlying internal object relations representing his sadism and aggression.

Although the patient's anxieties about his sadism and his inability to protect the vulnerable parts of himself and others from his aggression were clearly represented in the manifest content of his dream, this material was not affectively alive in the session. In DPHP, it is not uncommon for unconscious conflicts to present themselves early in treatment, often quite clearly, in dream material. Although it is worth commenting on the object relations and anxieties represented in the dream, we do not anticipate that these interpretations will lead to much more than intellectual understanding. It is only when the conflict is currently activated and being enacted in the patient's life and in the treatment that interpretation of a conflict will be meaningful and lead to insight.

TACTIC 4: ANALYZING THE RELATIONSHIP BETWEEN THE DOMINANT CONFLICT AND THE TREATMENT GOALS

We have covered the tactics the DPHP therapist uses to receive the patient's verbal and nonverbal communications, to identify a selected fact and a dominant conflict, to define that conflict in terms of the dominant object relations, and to systematically analyze the defensive and impulsive object relations associated with the identified conflict. At this point, we consider the role played by treatment goals in DPHP and the tactics employed to meet these goals as efficiently and effectively as possible.

As we have discussed, DPHP is a treatment organized around specific treatment goals agreed upon as part of the consultation process. In this sense, DPHP is a focused treatment, one that is oriented toward integration of conflictual object relations, with the aim of reducing personality rigidity in *circumscribed areas of functioning* defined by the patient's presenting complaints and treatment goals.

BRINGING CORE CONFLICTS INTO FOCUS BEFORE MAKING LINKS TO THE TREATMENT GOALS

DPHP relies on free and open communication and analysis of resistance from a position of technical neutrality in order to gain access to the patient's unconscious conflicts and internal object relations. To this end, the patient is encouraged to speak as freely and openly as possible, saying whatever comes to mind without censoring or pursuing any particular agenda. It should be evident that this approach is fundamentally incompatible with a focal approach, such as would be employed in a short-term dynamic psychotherapy. In short-term dynamic therapy, before beginning treatment the therapist instructs the patient to orient his comments around the focus of the treatment, and once treatment begins the therapist interprets the patient's deviation from the focus as resistance to adhering to the focal frame of the treatment. In contrast, in DPHP, the first tactical decision made in relation to the treatment goals is that the patient will focus on the exploration of his internal object relations and defensive operations as they are enacted in the treatment, without attention to treatment goals.

The second tactical decision in relation to treatment goals has to do with determining at what point the therapist should introduce discussion of the treatment goals. In DPHP, we begin by fully exploring a given conflict in the here and now, without attempting to link it to treatment goals or presenting problems. In this process, neither patient nor therapist is thinking, "How can I understand the patient's presenting problems?" Rather, the question is "How can I understand the conflicts presently being enacted in the treatment?" Up to this point, the treatment goals do not affect the therapist's tactical approach. *However, once a particular conflict has come into focus, the treatment goals become a prominent part of the therapist's thinking.* From then on, one of the therapist's tactics is to analyze the relationship between the dominant conflict being enacted in the treatment and the treatment goals.

Every patient has core or dominant conflicts that affect him in many areas of functioning. Some areas of functioning will be very powerfully and obviously affected by a given conflict, whereas others will be much more subtly affected. In DPHP, we focus on the patient's core conflicts as they pertain to those areas of impairment that are of greatest concern to him. We link the patient's dominant conflicts, as they come into focus in the treatment, with the patient's presenting complaints or with treatment goals as part of the process of interpretation and working through.

FOCUSING ON TREATMENT GOALS AS PART OF THE PROCESS OF WORKING THROUGH

As we have described, it is the process of working through that we believe leads to change in dynamic psychotherapy. In working through, a conflict is repeatedly enacted and analyzed in different contexts and from different perspectives, leading to an increasingly deep and complex understanding of the particular conflict and its links to other conflicts. In DPHP, the therapist preferentially emphasizes the patient's presenting complaints and treatment goals as a context for working through. As a conflict comes into focus, the therapist raises the question, "How might this conflict relate to the patient's presenting problems and the treatment goals?" As a conflict is repeatedly enacted during the course of the treatment, the therapist will have many opportunities to explore and interpret the relationship between that conflict and the treatment goals.

This tactic calls upon the therapist to make decisions about how to properly time and place appropriate emphasis on the link between the conflict currently dominant in the treatment and the treatment goals. At what point in the process of analyzing a particular conflict should the therapist introduce the treatment goals? How powerfully, at any given point, should the therapist emphasize the link between the dominant conflict and these goals?

WHEN TO BRING IN THE TREATMENT GOALS

There are implicit guideposts that experienced DPHP therapists use when deciding when and when not to make a link between dynamic material enacted and explored in a session and the patient's presenting complaints. First and foremost, the therapist always keeps in mind that his highest priority is to understand the patient's core conflicts. With this in mind, the therapist will analyze the conflictual object relations enacted in the treatment in their defensive functions until the core conflict comes into focus. In this process, the therapist does not select material or conflicts to explore, nor does the patient. The unfolding of the patient's conflicts is an organic part of the treatment.

It is only after a conflict and the associated object relations have been clearly described and explored that the therapist turns his mind to generating hypotheses about how the conflict may relate to the patient's presenting complaints. This effort is facilitated by the inevitable fact that whatever problems brought the patient to treatment will continue during the treatment. However, even after a conflict has come into focus and the therapist is ready to link the conflict in question to the treatment goals, he does not do this by raising the issue of the treatment goals out of the blue or by forcing the issue in an artificial fashion. Rather, the therapist keeps his eye open for situations in which the links to the treatment goals present themselves in a natural and meaningful way. The therapist waits for opportunities; he does not create them. In fact, sometimes it is less that the therapist chooses to focus on or pursue certain issues and more that he chooses to pursue others less actively.

To illustrate the tactical approach adopted by the DPHP therapist—that is, being open to all aspects of the patient's communications and at the same time streamlining his interventions to address specific treatment goals—let us return to the two patients whose treatments we have most recently discussed.

FIRST CLINICAL ILLUSTRATION OF FOCUSING ON THE TREATMENT GOALS

The single professional woman with conflicts around dependency whom we described earlier in this chapter (to illustrate the tactic of selecting a priority theme) presented to treatment after being jilted by a man she had been involved with for many years. In the aftermath of the relationship, the patient's former lover had emerged as manipulative and untrustworthy to a degree that she had never imagined. The patient came to treatment wanting to understand how she had chosen such a man, to get past the agonizing loss of the relationship, and to do whatever she needed to in order to be able to become involved with a more suitable man in the future. There is no question that the patient had other areas of difficulty where she had made compromises or was not necessarily functioning optimally, but her impairments were either relatively limited in those areas or not of particular concern to her.

For example, in her professional life, although the patient was extremely successful, she periodically failed to make important deadlines or to completely follow through on important initiatives, and her reputation had suffered to some degree as a result. Furthermore, in stressful moments, she had a tendency to lash out at the people working for her in a fashion that was somewhat inappropriate for the setting. She was satisfied with her friendships but was seen as something of a "taker" by those closest to her, and she was essentially estranged from her siblings. During the consultation process, the patient and therapist agreed that these additional areas of functioning were clearly impacted by her conflicts and could be successfully addressed if she chose to focus on these areas. However, the patient decided that she felt relatively comfortable in these areas and opted to focus on her romantic difficulties.

As the patient's conflicts came into focus, the therapist consistently linked them to her difficulties with intimacy and her previous choice of a man. For example, as more paranoid object relations that had been repressed emerged in the treatment and came to be understood, the therapist made a link between them and the patient's relationship with her former boyfriend. The therapist began by pointing out how the patient's fantasies about the dangers inherent in dependent relationships had been actualized in her relationship to her boyfriend. This intervention opened the door to the patient's exploring how her conflicts around dependency and envy had, out of her awareness, drawn her to a man with whom she could actually play out some of the things she most feared unconsciously.

At another point in the treatment, the patient came to understand and to take responsibility for the more exploitative and sadistic parts of herself as they were activated in dependent, intimate relationships. This object relation was explored, again in relation to the patient's choice of a man. Taking responsibility for exploitative parts of herself meant that she was no longer drawn to partners who enabled her to externalize those parts of herself. Furthermore, she no longer needed to protect herself from the possibility of a relationship based in genuine, mutual ("mature") dependency by selecting an unsuitable and untrustworthy partner. The therapist made many interpretations of this kind as the patient's conflictual object relations were brought into the treatment and were worked through. The therapist pointed out, for example, that maintaining a relationship with a man like her former boyfriend ultimately served to protect her from the pain of being sadistic in relation to someone she deeply loved and who was worthy of her love.

SECOND CLINICAL ILLUSTRATION OF FOCUSING ON THE TREATMENT GOALS

As another example, we return to the patient who came to treatment feeling like a loser, unable to assert himself or to actively pursue achievement of the power and monetary success he desired. This patient had other areas of difficulty apart from self-esteem and professional advancement. For example, he had long-standing sexual inhibitions that he chose not to address in the therapy. Also, he was perfectly happy to maintain a somewhat distant relationship with his wife, who also seemed satisfied with this arrangement. Finally, this patient was having difficulty coping with the demands of caring for his elderly parents. Any or all of these areas of difficulty could have been given priority in the treatment; however, the patient opted to focus on his conflicts around power in his professional life.

As the patient's conflicts came into focus, the therapist emphasized the links between the object relations being enacted and the patient's inhibitions in relation to power, authority, and money, while paying less attention to his inhibitions in relation to sexuality and intimacy. For example, as the patient's anxieties about his sadism came into focus, the therapist suggested that the patient was afraid to be in a position of power because he feared losing control and attacking people less powerful or more vulnerable than himself. Similarly, when the patient responded to personal and professional successes by feeling anxious or guilty, the therapist again emphasized the link to the patient's inhibitions in relation to money and success in the workplace. Although the therapist commented on the links between the patient's conflicts and his emotionally distanced and sexually inhibited relationship with his wife, these links were not emphasized in the process of working through. In sum, as a particular conflict came into focus, the therapist emphasized how this related to the patient's inhibitions with regard to pursuing professional and financial advancement and paid less attention to exploring how these same conflicts left the patient inhibited in other areas as well.

COMMENTS ON THE CLINICAL ILLUSTRATIONS

In the two clinical examples presented, the therapist began by bringing the patient's core conflicts into focus. The first patient's conflicts were primarily around dependency and intimacy, whereas the second patient's conflicts were primarily around power and sadism. In both cases, these conflicts impacted many aspects of the patient's functioning. This had been discussed during the consultation process, and the therapist and patient had agreed to focus on a particular area of difficulty of special concern to the patient. The first patient wanted to be able to have a satisfactory romantic relationship, and the second wanted to enjoy power and money. As the patients' core conflicts came into focus, the patients' therapists began to keep an eye out for the opportunity to link the conflicts being enacted to the treatment goals and presenting complaints.

The process of linking the patient's dominant conflicts to the treatment goals requires restraint on the part of the therapist. It is often tempting to prematurely bring in treatment goals before the dominant conflict has become sufficiently clear. In addition, some therapists find it difficult to pass up opportunities to pursue potential avenues of therapeutic benefit—for example, the first patient's inhibitions in the workplace or the second patient's sexual symptoms—simply because these areas of potential benefit are not part of the treatment goals. Although other areas of difficulty should be discussed and to some degree explored, the therapist should not emphasize them in the same way that he does the treatment goals.

AVOIDING THE TREATMENT GOALS

In practice, in DPHP, it generally happens quite naturally that the treatment goals receive more attention than do other areas of difficulty. This is because the patient is more likely to pick up on the therapist's interventions when they pertain to those areas of functioning that are of the greatest concern to him. If, for an extended period of time, the patient chooses to focus on areas other than the treatment goals, the therapist needs to assess whether this represents a change in the patient's priorities. If the patient's goals for the treatment *have* changed, this should be explicitly discussed, along with the question of whether the treatment goals should be revised.

If the patient's priorities have in fact not changed, the therapist should interpret the patient's avoidance of the treatment goals as a form of resistance. The therapist can point out that, for unclear reasons, the patient is choosing to avoid exploring his difficulties in those areas of functioning that are of greatest importance to him. It is assumed that this behavior is driven by anxiety of some sort that can be explored and ultimately understood in terms of the patient's conflicts. Invariably, exploration of the patient's anxiety with regard to focusing on the goals that he has selected for himself will have direct bearing on the dynamics and conflictual object relations underlying his presenting complaints and treatment goals.

Some patients will actively and consistently resist addressing the treatment goals over extended periods of time. These patients may discuss their core conflicts in depth but will consistently move away from or deflect the therapist's efforts to focus on the problem that brought them to treatment. This clinical situation calls upon the therapist to be quite active and persistent. The tactic here is first to call the patient's attention to his resistance to addressing the issues that brought him to treatment and help him explore his motivation for doing so. If the patient persists in dodging the therapist's interventions, the therapist can then follow up on his initial intervention by focusing on and exploring the ways in which the patient has rejected the therapist's efforts to bring in the treatment goals.

In response to the therapist's activity in such a situation, the patient may feel that the therapist is deviating from his usual role by "pushing too hard." Typically, the patient will experience the therapist's activity in a particular light—for example, feeling that the therapist is being critical, seductive, or rejecting of the patient. Indeed, it is not uncommon for the therapist to have complementary feelings—for example, to wonder if he is being too forceful or controlling of the session or is perhaps deviating from a position of neutrality in his activity. The challenge for the therapist is to contain his anxiety about pushing the patient and to restrain whatever inclination he may have to pull back and be passive. Instead, the therapist can—while maintaining a position of neutrality—actively help the patient explore his reactions to the therapist's activity. In this process, it will almost always emerge that some aspect of the patient's conflict has been enacted in the transference.

CLINICAL ILLUSTRATION OF A PATIENT'S AVOIDING THE TREATMENT GOALS

A 25-year-old graduate student came to treatment complaining of difficulties completing his doctoral thesis. The patient spent the first 6 months of therapy exploring his highly problematic relationship with a critical and rejecting father upon whom the patient was financially dependent. At the beginning of treatment, the patient had held an idealized view of his father and of their relationship. However, while still in the first few months of treatment, the patient began to develop a more complex and realistic view of his relationship with his father, one that acknowledged the mutual hostility between them.

Six months into treatment, the patient was feeling much better about himself, and he was getting along better with his live-in girlfriend. However, whenever the therapist raised the issue of the patient's dissertation, the patient would speak about it in general terms for a session or two and then move on to talk of other things. On the one hand, on the surface, the treatment seemed to be going well, and there was no question that the patient's conflicts with his father were closely tied to his difficulty with his dissertation. On the other hand, the therapist was aware that the patient avoided focusing on the dissertation in a way that would enable him to develop a deeper understanding of the specific issues involved. The therapist noted that, in the countertransference, he too had been tempted to lapse into a "goal-less" exploration of the patient's core conflicts.

Having reflected on this, the therapist decided to share his observations with the patient. He began by reminding the patient that he had come to treatment complaining of difficulty completing his academic requirement and that the goals of the treatment were organized around better understanding his difficulties in this area. The therapist then pointed out that, although they had covered many important issues in the therapy and the patient was clearly making gains, the topic of the dissertation had been largely neglected. The therapist went on to suggest that what was happening in the treatment mirrored what was happening in the patient's life—that is, everything seemed to be going well, but he was failing to advance professionally.

Rather than picking up on the therapist's comments in his usual, pleasant manner, the patient silently glared at the therapist. When they explored the patient's uncharacteristic silence and hostility, it emerged that he had had a very negative reaction to the therapist's comments. The patient explained, and complained, that the therapist was painfully letting him down by behaving exactly as his father did. Father and therapist seemed only to notice what the patient *failed* to do and cared only about his professional advancement, to the neglect of his happiness.

As he listened to the patient and weathered the patient's expressions of disappointment, criticism, and hostility, the therapist began to feel apologetic, as though he had hurt the patient. As he reflected on this reaction, it occurred to him that he had avoided confronting the patient sooner out of his own reluctance to leave the patient feeling misunderstood, critical, and angry.

The therapist identified the object relation enacted in the transference as one between a demanding, critical father who relentlessly pushed his son to succeed and a son who wanted to avoid conflict. The therapist noted to himself that this was the first time the patient had consciously experienced the therapist as anything like his father, and he was struck by how his efforts to "bring in the focus" had stimulated such a violent reaction in the patient; it was as though a latent transference had emerged full force when the therapist confronted the patient's resistance to addressing the goals of treatment. The therapist was also struck by the role reversal that quickly followed his intervention, and he reflected upon how, in the countertransference, as he weathered the patient's criticism, he likely had had a taste of how the patient felt when castigated by his father.

The patient and the therapist spent a number of sessions exploring what had been enacted in the treatment. Over time, both came to feel that, in some ways, the patient had been using the treatment to feel better without having to address his fears around success and competition. At the same time, the patient was passively rebelling against, while simultaneously maintaining dependence upon, a controlling father in the transference. Both the patient's rebellion and his dependence functioned to keep his identification with his father out of the treatment and also to keep his critical hostility out of the transference. This episode was the beginning of fruitful exploration of the patient's reluctance to use the treatment to address his anxieties about his dissertation and, ultimately, of his reluctance to complete it and to move on with his life.

WHAT HAPPENS TO THE PATIENT'S FUNCTIONING IN AREAS OUTSIDE THE TREATMENT GOALS?

Before closing this section, we address the question of what happens to the DPHP patient's functioning in those areas not included in the treatment goals. Returning to our two clinical illustrations, we are thinking of the single professional woman's maladaptive behavior in the workplace and the submissive male patient's inhibitions in relation to love and intimacy. These areas of difficulty, although not included in the treatment goals, are closely related to them insofar as they are manifestations of the same core conflicts. As a result, we often see some degree of improvement in areas of functioning that extend beyond those designated by the treatment goals, as part of a ripple effect. In general, the less severe the patient's personality rigidity, the more likely we are to see therapeutic benefits in areas of functioning not included in the treatment goals. In patients with greater degrees of personality rigidity, however, the gains made in areas outside the treatment goals are often far less robust than those made in relation to the treatment goals themselves. The fact that the treatment has not ameliorated or even addressed all of the patient's difficulties is a reality that will be confronted and worked through during the termination phase of every DPHP treatment.

SUGGESTED READINGS

Busch F: The ego and its significance in analytic interventions. J Am Psychoanal Assoc 44:1073–1099, 1996

Fenichel O: Problems of Psychoanalytic Technique. New York, Psychoanalytic Quarterly, 1941

Levy ST, Inderbitzin LB: Interpretation, in The Technique and Practice of Psychoanalysis, Vol 2. Edited by Sugarman A, Nemiroff RA, Greenson DP. Madison, CT, International Universities Press, 1992, pp 101–116

PATIENT ASSESSMENT, PHASES OF TREATMENT, AND COMBINING DPHP WITH OTHER TREATMENTS

9

PATIENT ASSESSMENT AND DIFFERENTIAL TREATMENT PLANNING

Patient assessment and treatment planning make up the *consultation* phase of dynamic psychotherapy for higher level personality pathology (DPHP). Patient assessment involves characterizing the patient's 1) presenting symptoms and pathological personality traits, 2) general personality functioning, and 3) level of personality organization. A comprehensive diagnostic assessment, including DSM-IV-TR Axis I and Axis II diagnosis and structural diagnosis, paves the way for treatment planning. Differential treatment planning involves 1) sharing diagnostic impressions with the patient, 2) defining treatment goals, 3) describing treatment options and their relative risks and benefits, and 4) helping the patient come to an informed decision with regard to how to proceed—a decision that reflects the patient's personal goals and needs and the therapist's expertise.

It is often possible to complete the consultative process in a single 1½-hour interview. However, many clinicians prefer to have the patient return for a second, 45-minute session to complete discussion of treatment planning.

A second meeting with the patient in consultation has the advantage of allowing patient and therapist time to reflect on the initial interview and then to use the second meeting to address aspects of the patient's internal and external situation that may have been omitted or inadequately explored in the initial consultation. In addition, a second meeting provides opportunity to explore the patient's reactions to the initial interview. Some patients, especially those with more complex problems or those about whom there is diagnostic uncertainty, may require two follow-up sessions after the initial meeting in order for the consultation to be completed and a treatment plan determined.

PATIENT ASSESSMENT AND THE DIAGNOSTIC INTERVIEW

In our approach to patient assessment, presenting symptoms and pathological personality traits are conceptualized as embedded in a particular personality organization. In our diagnostic interview, presenting symptoms and pathological personality traits are clearly characterized, leading to a descriptive diagnosis, and personality organization is explored in depth, leading to a structural diagnosis. Our interview is directive—asking specific questions of the patient and relying heavily on clarification of, and to some degree confrontation of, the patient's communications—and it focuses on the here and now, both the patient's current life situation and his current interactions with the interviewer, in contrast to the developmental past.

For purpose of clarity and economy, we divide our discussion of patient assessment into two parts (Table 9–1). First, we outline the data that our interview is designed to provide, describing the information that the clinician should have in order to make a diagnosis. Next, we outline the method whereby data are collected, which is derived from Kernberg's Structural Interview (Kernberg 1984).

DIAGNOSTIC INTERVIEW: THE DATA

DESCRIPTIVE DIAGNOSIS

Patient assessment begins with identification and characterization of the symptoms and pathological personality traits that brought the patient to treatment, followed by a thorough and systematic evaluation of all symptoms. This portion of the consultation involves data collection that would be part of any general psychiatric assessment. If there is a history of prior treatment, medication, and/or hospitalization, this information is reviewed, as are the patient's medical history, history of substance misuse, and family history of psychiatric illness.

With the patient's difficulties having been characterized, the next phase of the consultation is devoted to exploring the patient's personality, focusing on the degree to which symptoms and pathological personality traits interfere with personality functioning. To what degree do the patient's symptoms and pathological personality traits interfere with his relationships? Does he have a partner? Is he or has he ever been in love? What is the nature of his closest relationships? If he has children, what is the nature of his relationships with them? Does he have friends, and has he maintained friendships over time?

We also ask about work functioning. Does the patient have a career? If not, why not and does he have realistic career goals? Is his level of employment consistent with his level of education and his abilities? Does he do well at his job? Does he obtain satisfaction from his work? Does he get along well with or develop interpersonal problems with peers, bosses, and/or employees?

Finally, we ask about personal interests and what the patient does with his free time. Does he have activities he is invested in or has stayed with over time? Does he derive pleasure from his leisure time?

Having accumulated this information, the consultant has the information needed to make or to rule out a DSM-IV-TR Axis I and Axis II diagnosis.

STRUCTURAL DIAGNOSIS: ASSESSING PERSONALITY ORGANIZATION

There can be a fair amount of variability within a particular descriptive diagnostic category with regard to severity of personality pathology. (For example, some patients with histrionic personality disorder have only mild pathology of identity and object relations and function quite well, whereas others have pathology that is more severe and disruptive of functioning.) Therefore, diagnostic assessment will focus on structural as well as descriptive aspects of personality functioning.

TABLE 9–1. Patient assessment

The data: content domains

    Presenting symptoms and pathological personality traits

    General personality functioning

    Level of personality organization/structural diagnosis

The method: sources of information

    Psychiatric history

    Nonverbal communication

    Clarification and confrontation

    Countertransference

TABLE 9–2. Structural assessment of personality

	No personality pathology	Higher level personality pathology	Severe personality disorders
Level of personality organization	Normal personality organization	Neurotic level of personality organization or transition between neurotic and borderline levels of personality organization	Borderline level of personality organization
Sense of self and others	Sense of self and others well integrated, stable, and realistic	Sense of self and others relatively well integrated, stable, and realistic	Sense of self and others poorly integrated, superficial, unstable, and unrealistic
Quality of object relations	Capacity to appreciate needs of others independent of needs of the self	Capacity to appreciate needs of others independent of needs of the self	Need-fulfilling working model of relationships predominates
	Stable and deep interpersonal relations	Stable and deep, but possibly conflictual, interpersonal relations	Unstable and superficial interpersonal relations
	Sexual intimacy combined with tenderness	Difficulty integrating sexuality and tenderness	Severe impairment in love relations with absence of or chaotic sexual relations
Investments	Investments in work and leisure activities	Investments in work and/or leisure activities	Poor or absent investments in work and leisure activities
Defenses	Mature defenses predominate, variable neurotic defenses	Neurotic defenses predominate, variable mature and splitting-based defenses	Splitting-based defenses predominate
Rigidity	Flexibility	Rigidity	Severe rigidity
Reality testing	Intact and stable	Intact and stable	Essentially intact but deteriorates in the setting of affective intensity
Internalized value system	Fully developed and internalized value systems with flexible standards	Fully developed and internalized value systems but with excessively rigid standards	Contradictory and incompletely internalized value systems

As described in Chapter 2 ("A Psychodynamic Approach to Personality Pathology"), from a structural perspective, patients with higher level personality pathology fall into Kernberg's neurotic level of personality organization or into the transitional range between neurotic and borderline levels of personality organization. Dimensions of personality functioning evaluated as part of structural assessment are summarized in Table 9–2. We remind the reader that even though relevant dimensions of personality functioning are represented categorically in Table 9–2, they are in fact continuous.

Although we recommend systematic evaluation of personality organization, the experienced interviewer can often make an assessment of identity consolidation on the basis of his overall subjective experience during the interview. Specifically, the integrated internal experience of the patient with higher level personality pathology will lend clarity and relatively easy comprehensibility to the interpersonal reality and past history that the patient presents, and it will be relatively easy for the interviewer to empathize with the patient, his conflicts, and his description of significant others. In contrast, while the patient with more severe personality pathology may increase his more realistic behavior during the interview, he simultaneously makes plain the emptiness, chaos, and confusion in his life situation and object relations, leaving the interviewer with a sense of confusion and incomplete understanding and making it difficult for the interviewer to empathize with the patient and his significant others.

IDENTITY: SENSE OF SELF AND SENSE OF OTHERS

When assessing a patient who presents with personality pathology in the setting of relatively intact reality testing (i.e., a psychotic disorder has been ruled out), the clinician will focus on clinical features that reflect identity consolidation versus identity pathology to distinguish between higher level and more severe personality pathology. In particular we evaluate the degree to which the individual's sense of himself and significant others is complex, realistic, and stable versus superficial or polarized, unrealistic, and unstable. To a lesser degree, identity formation will also be reflected in the degree to which an individual has the capacity to invest in long-term professional and personal goals and values and in intimate love and sexual relationships.

When seen in consultation, patients with consolidated identity are able to provide information about themselves with subtlety and depth in a way that permits the interviewer to rapidly gain knowledge about many areas of the patient's life. During an 1½ hour–long consultation, the interviewer will easily develop a progressively clear and detailed impression of the patient's internal experience and external functioning, including both strengths and weakness, that is consistent with the interviewer's overall impression of the patient. In the patient with consolidated identity, apparent distortions in self-perception or self-presentation and poorly integrated aspects of self experience will be limited to specific areas of conflict; for example, a successful patient may not appreciate that he is valued by his employers, or a serious and otherwise responsible professional may routinely endanger his reputation by visiting prostitutes while traveling on business. Similarly, as the patient describes his relationships with others, the important people in the patient's life will emerge as three-dimensional, realistic, understandable, and complex individuals.

In contrast, the patient with poorly consolidated identity is likely to leave the interviewer with a vague or confused sense of the patient's functioning in various aspects of his daily life. The information that the patient provides about himself will typically be vague, superficial, and internally inconsistent, so that it is difficult for the interviewer to develop a clear impression of the patient's internal experience or external functioning. For example, a patient may describe himself as chronically suicidal and overwhelmed by anxiety, yet in the next sentence maintain that he has a highly successful professional life, or he may describe himself as "very outgoing and social," even though he has no friends in the city in which he lives. Similarly, in the setting of identity pathology, the patient's descriptions of the people in his world tend to be superficial and poorly differentiated, "black and white" or caricature-like, and internally inconsistent.

QUALITY OF INTERNAL AND EXTERNAL OBJECT RELATIONS

When we inquire about quality of object relations, we are interested in the patient's conception of the basic nature of close relationships and his capacity to appreciate and care about the needs and feelings of others. Does he see relationships in terms of need fulfillment, by which we mean in terms of who gets what from the relationship and which person gets more, or does he have a sense of a mutual give and take? The stable and integrated sense of self and others seen in patients with consolidated identity is associated with a capacity for object relations characterized by concern for the needs of others, independent of the needs of the self; the capacity for mutual give and take; and the capacity to depend on others, as well as to be depended upon. Interpersonal relationships are stable in quality and sustained over time, marked by trust and respect for the other as an individual. To the degree that there is disruption of interpersonal functioning, it is limited to specific areas of conflict.

In contrast, identity pathology is typically associated with a need-fulfilling view of relationships in which the patient conceptualizes relationships in terms of how much he gets and how much he gives, and a limited ability to care about the needs of others independent of his own needs and wishes. In the patient with severe personality pathology, close interpersonal relationships are typically unstable, often chaotic, colored by mistrust and hostility, and lacking in intimacy.

DEFENSES AND PERSONALITY RIGIDITY

In the severe personality disorders, image-distorting, or splitting-based, defenses affect the patient's behavior and also lead to distortion and instability of interpersonal experience. As a result, the predominance of splitting-based defenses characteristic of the patient with severe personality pathology is typically relatively easy to spot during the course of a diagnostic interview. The polarized and unstable sense of self and others and the contradictory personality traits (e.g., a demure elementary school teacher who earns extra cash by working as a stripper) that are often core features of the severe personality disorders reflect the impact of splitting-based defensive operations on the patient's internal experience and external functioning. In addition, during the consultation, the patient with identity pathology will typically employ defensive operations that involve controlling the interviewer in one way or another; in particular, projective identification, omnipotent control, and idealization/devaluation can be identified in the countertransference in conjunction with evaluation of a patient with severe personality pathology.

In contrast, the defenses of the patient with higher level personality pathology can be more difficult to identify in a diagnostic interview because they are less likely to affect the patient's behavior or the interviewer's experience. As a result, we tend to infer rather than observe the predominance of neurotic defenses when we see personality rigidity in conjunction with a consolidated stable, integrated, and realistic sense of self and others. As described in Chapter 2, personality rigidity will be reflected in a history of repetitive, maladaptive behavior patterns that the patient is either unaware of or unable to change. In the interview, maladaptive personality traits, such as an excessive need to please or a need to feel in control, will be enacted in the patient's interactions with the interviewer.

ETHICAL FUNCTIONING

In addition to examining identity and defenses, when assessing personality organization, we evaluate the patient's ethical functioning (Kernberg 1984). This assessment is typically less important in patients with higher level personality pathology, with whom we see relatively well integrated and stable internalized value systems and moral functioning; pathology of ethical functioning in patients with higher level personality pathology typically manifests as inflexibility and is often characterized by a tendency toward excessive self-criticism and unduly high internal standards.

In contrast, in patients with identity pathology, moral functioning is more variable—value systems are not fully internalized, and pathology of moral functioning is common (Kernberg 1984). Pathology of morality in patients with identity pathology frequently manifests as a combination of excessively harsh or rigid moral functioning that coexists with ego-syntonic "lacunae" or deficits in other areas of moral functioning (e.g., a member of the clergy is devoted to service of God and community but comfortably exploits others for personal gain). In practice, the presence of antisocial behavior patterns and their relative severity reflect the degree of pathology of the patient's internalized ethical and value systems. In an evaluation of the patient with severe personality pathology, the assessment of ethical functioning becomes an important consideration in differential treatment planning and prognosis (Clarkin et al. 2006).

DIAGNOSTIC INTERVIEW: THE METHOD

When assessing a patient, the psychodynamic clinician does not rely solely on what the patient tells the interviewer about himself. In addition, the interviewer pays close attention to the patient's behavior, the patient's interactions with the interviewer, and the way the patient makes the interviewer feel in the countertransference. To deepen his understanding of the patient's personality organization and personality rigidity, the interviewer will ask for *clarification* of the patient's subjective experience when information is vague, unclear, or apparently missing, and he will gently point out omissions (*confrontation*) in the patient's narrative or inconsistencies in his verbal and nonverbal communications. Specifically, the interviewer will ask the patient how he understands these inconsistencies and how he feels about them, and the interviewer will encourage the patient to provide additional information that might clarify what has been occurring.

At the same time, the consultant will pay close attention to how the patient responds to these interventions. Typically, interventions of this kind will lead to further activation of the patient's defensive operations and amplification of their expression in the patient's interactions with the interviewer, where they can be further explored. This sequence challenges the patient to reflect on and explore his behaviors and motivations, and provides the interviewer with the opportunity to evaluate the patient's capacity to do so. In the end, the consultant will combine what he hears about the

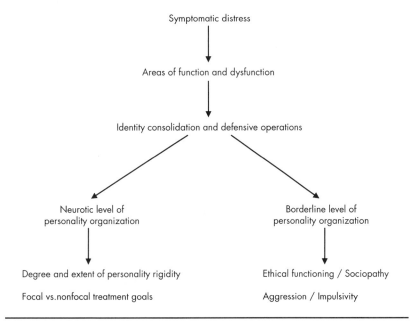

FIGURE 9-1. Decision tree for patient assessment.

patient's subjective experience and what he observes in the patient's behavior and interactions with him during the interview, in order to make inferences about the patient's level of personality organization.

The clinical assessment can be conceptualized as a decision tree (Figure 9–1). At each level of inquiry, information is acquired and used to generate hypotheses that will guide and focus the clinician's approach at the next level of inquiry.

ASSESSMENT OF PRESENTING PROBLEMS, PERSONALITY FUNCTIONING, AND LEVEL OF PERSONALITY ORGANIZATION

The Structural Interview

The Structural Interview, developed by Kernberg (1984), is a clinical interview that can be administered by an experienced clinician in approximately 90 minutes. The interview is designed to distinguish borderline personality organization from neurotic personality organization, on the one hand, and subtle forms of psychosis, on the other, while at the same time obtaining the sort of descriptive information about symptoms and personality traits provided by a general psychiatric interview.

The Structural Interview is loosely structured and relies on the clinical judgment and skill of the interviewer. It focuses on the patient's symptoms and pathological personality traits, difficulties associated with them, the patient's capacity to reflect on his difficulties, and the particular ways in which his problems are manifested in his interactions with the interviewer. In the interview, the consultant will periodically diverge from exploring the patient's difficulties and the nature of his relationships with significant others in order to make use of clarification and confrontation, employed to highlight and explore the defensive operations and conflictual issues activated in the patient–interviewer interaction. This process provides the interviewer with additional data that will complement what the patient provides in his narrative, and will enable the clinician to rule out psychotic illness and to pursue the differential diagnosis of neurotic versus borderline level of personality organization.

This approach, of obtaining information about present difficulties and functioning while periodically confronting the patient's defensive operations, enables the interviewer to highlight the descriptive pathology with which the patient presents while simultaneously assessing underlying personality organization.

Phase I. The Structural Interview begins with inquiries about the patient's presenting difficulties. The interviewer begins with a request for information, saying something like, "Please tell me what brought you to this interview. What is the nature of your difficulties and what are your expectations as to how treatment might be of help to you?" This opening provides the patient opportunity to discuss his symptoms, his chief reasons for coming to treatment, and any other difficulties he is experiencing in his present life. In listening to the patient, the interviewer can assess the patient's awareness of his pathology, his appreciation of the need for treatment, and the degree to which his expectations of treatment are realistic or unrealistic. Failures of reality testing and thought disorders will typically become apparent quickly, as the patient struggles (or fails to struggle) to answer this complex, abstract, and unstructured request for information. Further, patients with identity diffusion will often identify themselves by responding to the initial inquiry with apparently thoughtless and chaotic presentation of their difficulties, life situation, and expectations for treatment.

If the patient responds to the initial request for information in a fashion that is easy to follow and understand, clearly describing his symptoms and presenting problems and responding appropriately to the interviewer's request for clarification, the first part of the interview will closely resemble a general psychiatric interview. In contrast, if the patient's responses to these early inquiries and/or his behavior in the interview are poorly organized, peculiar, or confusing, the interviewer accordingly will focus attention in this area.

The goal here is to distinguish between a patient with psychotic illness, on the one hand, and a patient with identity pathology, on the other. The interviewer will begin by pointing out areas of vagueness or contradiction, asking for clarification, and inquiring as to whether the patient can understand the interviewer's confusion. In response to this sort of intervention, patients with identity diffusion will typically become more anxious but will also be able to respond to the interviewer's questions and to empathize with his confusion, and will commonly become better organized in the process. In contrast, patients with psychotic disorders will have difficulty following the line of inquiry and understanding the interviewer's confusion, while becoming increasingly disorganized.

Phase II. After the presenting difficulties have been described and explored and (if applicable) a psychotic process has been ruled out, the next phase of the Structural Interview involves inquiring about the patient's personality. The interviewer can begin with a statement such as, "I have gotten a pretty clear sense of the symptoms and difficulties that bring you to treatment. Can you tell me now about how you function in your daily life, and about the ways in which your difficulties have or have not interfered with your functioning?"

If, when presenting further data about himself, the patient conveys information that the interviewer cannot put together in his mind—particularly contradictory data that do not fit with the internal image of the patient and his life that the interviewer is building up—the possibility of a diagnosis of identity pathology is raised. This is another juncture in the interview at which tactful probing of potential or apparent contradictions is indicated, to evaluate the extent to which contradictory self-images are present, or the extent to which the patient presents a solid, well-integrated conception of himself. The goal is to distinguish between higher level personality pathology, in which conflictual aspects of functioning are split off from a central self experience, and identity diffusion, in which there is a globally dissociated quality of self experience. In practice, this distinction is generally made quite easily.

In patients with higher level personality pathology, while we frequently come upon peripheral areas of self experience that are contradictory, they are split off from and contradictory to a well-integrated, central area of subjective experience attached to a dominant and stable sense of self. Thus, while we do not expect total harmony in the patient with higher level personality pathology, we do expect to see a central subjective integration of the self-concept, which the therapist can use to empathize with the patient and to construct an internal

image of the patient in his mind. In this context, when one explores contradictory areas of experience or functioning, it becomes clear that the patient experiences these as ego alien, or "ego dystonic," and that they are seen as not fitting
into his otherwise integrated picture of himself. This sort of information often
serves as a window into the patient's conflicts and/or interpersonal difficulties,
but such a situation is different from that seen in identity diffusion, in which
there is no integrated, central, and dominant self experience.

In contrast, when we explore areas of apparent contradiction in the communications from patients with significant identity pathology, we can identify multiple contradictory aspects of functioning and self experience in the
absence of an underlying or central sense of self. These patients are well
aware that their self experience is inconsistent, internally contradictory, and
often chaotic. In fact, it is common for patients with clinically significant
identity pathology, when confronted with areas of inconsistency, to complain of not having an authentic, stable, or integrated sense of self, or of confusion about which aspects of their internal experience are "really me."

Phase III.   The final step in the structural interview is to acquire whatever
additional information may still be needed to clarify the nature of the patient's
identity consolidation. Typically, much of the information needed to determine the patient's level of personality organization will have been provided in
the course of exploring the nature of the patient's difficulties and personality
functioning. For example, in the setting of describing recurrent problems with
employers, a patient will provide the interviewer with information about the
patient's representations of others in areas of conflict. Similarly, listening to
the patient describe his chronic marital and sexual difficulties, the interviewer
can gain information about the quality of the patient's object relations.

However, to learn more about the patient's inner experience and to
identify more subtle forms of identity pathology as well as better integrated
narcissistic pathology, it is helpful at this point in the interview to directly
evaluate the degree of integration of the patient's sense of self and his sense
of others. The interviewer might introduce this phase of the interview by
saying something like, "At this point, I would like to shift gears a bit, to hear
more about you as a person, the way you perceive yourself, the way you feel
others perceive you, anything you think might be helpful for me to get a
real feeling for you as a person."

This statement calls on the patient to self-reflect as well as to present
an integrated view of his internal experience and his external functioning.
As a result, patients with identity pathology will have particular difficulty
responding to this line of inquiry. When the patient has difficulty, the interviewer should prompt the patient, encouraging him to broaden and

deepen his description of himself, for example, by pointing out that the patient seems to be emphasizing the things he is good at, and are there areas in which he faces more difficulty? Or perhaps by pointing out that the patient has done a good job of describing how others see him but has said little about how he feels about himself inside.

Having explored the degree of integration of the patient's sense of self, the interviewer can for the last time revisit the patient's experience of the important people in his world. In this phase of the interview, we focus on the patient's most intimate relationships, because in patients with severe personality disorders—who lack a stable and integrated picture of the people in their lives—deficits in the patient's sense of others are typically most pronounced with the people who are important to the patient. In addition, better integrated narcissistic patients who have a relatively stable sense of self can be clearly identified at this point in the interview by virtue of the absence of subtlety and depth in their descriptions of others, findings that are most dramatic when the patient is describing the people with whom he is most closely involved.

The interviewer can open this phase of the inquiry by saying something along the lines of, "I would now like to ask you to tell me something about the people who are most important in your present life. Could you tell me something about them in such a way that, given our limited time here, I might form a real, live impression of them?" If the patient is having difficulty, the interviewer can prompt him by specifically asking the patient to identify the person to whom he is closest, and then inviting the patient to describe the person, as he might if he were writing a paragraph about him in a story.

Narcissistic pathology.   It is in the exploration of the degree of integration of the patient's sense of others and the degree of pathology in his object relations that narcissistic pathology can be diagnosed most easily. This is because patients with narcissistic personality disorder can present with difficulties related to personality rigidity in the setting of a relatively stable sense of self, making it difficult at times in the early phases of the interview to distinguish a patient with a narcissistic personality disorder from a patient with higher level personality pathology. However, in this, the final phase of the interview, in which the patient is invited to describe the people close to him, the patient with narcissistic pathology will provide descriptions of others strikingly lacking in subtlety and depth, to a degree grossly inconsistent with the patient's apparently high level of functioning and stable sense of self. This finding will typically be foreshadowed earlier in the interview in the context of exploring the patient's object relations, which are explicitly viewed in terms of need fulfillment in the narcissistic personality.

Past history.   Once we have a clear picture of the patient's presenting difficulties, personality functioning, and level of personality organization, we inquire briefly about his past as it relates to his current difficulties. Here, we obtain information about the patient's developmental history and current and past relationships with parents and siblings. In patients with higher level personality pathology, information regarding the patient's past follows naturally from exploration of his present personality. In this setting, the patient's description of his history and of his family of origin will deepen the interviewer's understanding of the patient and will typically enable the interviewer to develop preliminary hypotheses about the nature and origins of the patient's conflicts.

In contrast, in the patient with identity pathology, information about the past is generally sufficiently contaminated by the patient's present personality difficulties that it becomes difficult to know how to make use of the information the patient provides; the patient's descriptions of his past are as chaotic, confusing, and internally contradictory as are his descriptions of his current life. As a result, in patients with severe personality pathology, careful assessment of the patient's present life, identity consolidation, and quality of object relations provides the data necessary for assessment of personality pathology, and it is preferable to explore the past only along general lines, without trying to clarify or confront the patient's characterizations of his past experiences.

CLINICAL ILLUSTRATION OF ASPECTS OF THE STRUCTURAL INTERVIEW

Ms. P. was a petite, 32-year-old woman with shoulder-length hair, pleasant in appearance though somewhat nondescript, and dressed in casual clothes and wearing no makeup. She appeared younger than her stated age. She made good eye contact with the interviewer and answered his questions in a thoughtful fashion.

In response to the consultant's initial inquiry, Ms. P. explained that over the previous three months, she had found herself feeling "down." She had no good explanation for this. A close friend had greatly benefited from psychotherapy, and Ms. P. explained that she was curious about whether she could be helped as well.

In the interview, Ms. P.'s mood was reactive, and her affect was of full range. There were no neurovegetative symptoms of depression and no impaired functioning as a result of her low mood. There was no prior history of depression. When the interviewer asked Ms. P. what, if anything, had changed in her life about 3 months ago, Ms. P. responded that her fiancé had moved to the city in which Ms. P. lived, and they had moved in together. Ms. P. added that there was no reason why this would have left her feeling depressed; she was happy and comfortable with her relationship with her boyfriend.

Once the consultant felt that he had fully characterized Ms. P.'s presenting symptoms, he asked how, if at all, her depressed mood had been affecting her functioning in her professional and social life. Ms. P. responded that she was an actress, that she had been going to auditions, and that, lately, she had found herself feeling excessively inhibited when auditioning. She explained that this had always been a problem to some degree but that recently she had been having more difficulty than usual.

The interviewer had heard almost nothing so far in the interview about Ms. P.'s professional life. He was somewhat surprised to learn that Ms. P. was an actress, and his initial reaction was to think of Ms. P. as pursuing a career for which she seemed poorly suited; he found it difficult to see this self-contained and somewhat nondescript young woman as someone likely to succeed as a performer.

The interviewer asked Ms. P. whether she was currently working and how she supported herself. Ms. P. responded that she was currently unemployed. She had been in a television series for the past 2 years but had chosen not to renew her contract in order to pursue a longtime dream of working in the theatre. It was in this context that she was finding it difficult to audition.

As he inquired further about Ms. P.'s professional history, it gradually dawned on the interviewer that she was something of a celebrity. In fact, the consultant had on occasion seen the television series that Ms. P. described, an innovative and successful program popular with teenage viewers, and he now could identify Ms. P. as the hip young woman who was the central character in the show. As the interviewer tried to understand his somewhat confused response to Ms. P., he recognized that his attitude reflected not simply the way she told her story—omitting details that would have allowed him to appreciate the level of her professional accomplishments earlier in the interview—but also her somewhat inhibited and girlish self-presentation, which seemed inconsistent with star status as well as with the role she played so convincingly on television.

At this point, Ms. P. went on to explain that the problem she was having in auditions was in fact a large part of why she had decided to call upon the consultant; even though the people she was auditioning for were familiar with her name and her work, she found herself acting like a girlish newcomer in her auditions. The consultant asked further questions and ascertained that Ms. P. did not feel anxious working in front of cameras or live audiences but had always had some difficulty auditioning. She felt her problem had recently become more pronounced, and she believed her behavior was likely to undermine her opportunity to get the parts she wanted.

The interviewer asked for details (*clarification*) of Ms. P.'s experience when auditioning and the particular circumstances that made her anxious. She explained that she was clearly much more anxious auditioning for work in the theatre than she had been working in television. Television had been a compromise, and auditioning for jobs in the theatre felt much more highly charged. In addition, she was aware that she had most difficulty auditioning for male directors whom she especially admired and who were well respected in the industry. What was most striking to her was that the men she was most uncomfortable with were the ones who she knew saw her as talented and as someone they would like to work with. With these men, she felt as though she were "shrinking" when she walked into the audition, just when she most wanted to shine. She felt that in the end, she appeared foolish; it was very frustrating. She had walked out of her last audition feeling humiliated.

The consultant moved on to inquire further about Ms. P.'s romantic and social life; she described a 5-year relationship with her present boyfriend. They had a mutually supportive and pleasurable relationship, though Ms. P. felt that she and her boyfriend often seemed more like siblings than lovers. Ms. P. added that she felt that both of them were somewhat sexually inhibited. When the consultant inquired further, it emerged that she had had more passionate encounters with men to whom she felt less emotionally attached but that she viewed her sexual relationship with her boyfriend as satisfactory.

Ms. P. had several friends working in the theater and another group of friends from college now living in the same city as she. She was generally content with her life situation; she just wanted to be able to relax and enjoy things more, and, most of all, to feel more comfortable and behave more appropriately in her auditions.

By this point, the consultant felt it quite likely that Ms. P. presented with personality rigidity in the setting of higher level personality pathology and a relatively well consolidated identity. This diagnostic impression was consistent with the thoughtful and organized way in which she presented herself and her difficulties, the apparent stability and depth of her intimate and social relationships and her capacity to commit herself to a career. In addition, the consultant's personal reaction to her—one of growing respect and admiration, along with a sense of deepening understanding of her personality and her conflicts—was consistent with higher level personality pathology.

At the same time, the interviewer was struck by the apparent dissociation between, on the one hand, Ms. P.'s professional success and the way she behaved and felt when performing and, on the other hand, the way she felt and acted in auditions and to some degree had acted with the interviewer as well. The interviewer wanted to assess whether this inconsistency reflected conflicts around exhibitionism and competition split off from a dominant self, or whether Ms. P.'s difficulties were manifestations of mild identity pathology. The interviewer shared with her his difficulty in putting together how she could be so comfortable performing in front of a full theater, even when alone on stage, with how uncomfortable and inhibited she felt in auditioning for a small group.

Ms. P. agreed that this was perplexing, and she told the consultant that it was something she had tried hard to make sense of herself, but to no avail. Further, she had worked with her agent and with her manager, unsuccessfully, to feel more self-confident in her auditions. With regard to specific triggers for her girlish behavior, the only thing she had been able to identify was the connection between her anxiety and auditioning for powerful men whom she admired. She added that it probably was "some kind of father thing."

To further deepen his understanding of Ms. P., her conflicts, and her view of herself, the interviewer asked her to describe herself. Ms. P. responded that she thought of herself as a down-to-earth person, with good values, and said that she was caring and conscientious. As a younger person, she had had serious problems with self-esteem, and she had often found herself taking a back seat in relation to her more outgoing friends. Though no longer shy, Ms. P. felt that even now, her view of herself had not kept pace with her accomplishments.

When asked what she meant by this, Ms. P. explained that, though she understood she had a successful career and her name was well known, she did not feel accomplished. Further, she still had a tendency to see herself as in the shadow of others; only when she was performing did she see herself as worthy of special attention. The consultant asked Ms. P. if she saw herself as a competitive person. She responded that she did not, though she was aware that others often felt competitive with her, and recently she had begun to feel that perhaps she was more competitive than she liked to acknowledge.

The consultant felt that he had a clear sense of Ms. P.'s complaints, her personality, and her personality organization. She presented with feelings of depression in the absence of affective illness, possibly meeting criteria for an adjustment reaction. Recent stressors included leaving television to pursue her ambition to work on the stage and moving in with her boyfriend. She did not meet criteria for a DSM-IV-TR personality disorder. Her presenting complaints reflected personality rigidity organized around a defensive self-presentation in which she felt and acted like a self-deprecating girl. She presented with problems with self-esteem and conflicts around exhibitionism and competition embedded in a neurotic level of personality organization.

Ending the Assessment of Presenting Problems, Personality Functioning, and Level of Personality Organization

Once assessment of presenting problems, personality functioning, and level of personality organization has been completed, we come to a branch in the diagnostic decision tree (Figure 9–1). If the patient has a relatively well consolidated identity, the next step in the assessment process is to evaluate the severity of the patient's personality rigidity. In higher level personality pathology, it is severity of personality rigidity, in conjunction with the patient's motivation for and expectations of treatment, that will be important in guiding treatment planning. If the patient presents with significant identity pathology, the next step is to evaluate the patient's ethical functioning and the extent to which pathological aggression infiltrates personality functioning. For discussion of assessment of the patient with severe personality pathology, we refer the reader to Clarkin, Yeomans, and Kernberg (2006).

We should note here that, before ending the assessment phase of the consultation, it is helpful to ask the patient if there are things that have been left out or insufficiently covered in the interview that are important for the interviewer to know about him.

Assessment of Severity of Personality Rigidity

Once the diagnosis of higher level personality pathology has been made, the next step is to assess the severity of the patient's personality rigidity. Severity of personality rigidity can be conceptualized across three, to some degree overlapping, dimensions (Table 9–3):

TABLE 9–3. Assessment of severity of personality rigidity

How rigid are the patient's maladaptive personality traits?
(Relatively flexible—Highly inflexible)

How extreme are the patient's maladaptive personality traits?
(Mildly maladaptive or noticeable—Highly maladaptive and inappropriate)

How global are the patient's maladaptive personality traits?
(Relatively focal, affecting one major area of functioning—Infiltrating all areas of functioning)

---

1. *Degree of rigidity*, spanning a range from relatively flexible at the least severe end of the spectrum, to highly inflexible at the other
2. *Degree to which rigidity is maladaptive*, spanning a range from mildly maladaptive or mildly inappropriate personality traits at one end of the spectrum, through highly maladaptive and highly inappropriate personality traits at the other
3. *Degree to which rigidity globally affects personality functioning*, spanning from relatively focal manifestations of personality rigidity that adversely affect primarily one area of functioning at the least severe end of the spectrum, through global personality rigidity in which maladaptive personality traits adversely affect many or even all core areas of functioning

When personality rigidity is highly *inflexible*, the patient will report that he is unable to override or alter his maladaptive behavior patterns, even when he is fully aware of them and makes an effort to change. So, for example, Ms. P., the actress described in the previous section, was unable to change how she felt inside and how she behaved interpersonally in her auditions, no matter how hard she tried and no matter how many times she demonstrated to herself that her girlish attitude was uncalled for. In contrast, if her personality rigidity had been less inflexible, she would have been able to modify her behavior in auditions, perhaps by practicing being more assertive or by getting advice from friends. Even though she might still have felt like a small child internally, if her personality traits had been less rigid, she would have been able to modify her behavior so that it was more appropriate.

When personality rigidity is highly *maladaptive*, the behavior patterns that the patient is unable to change are highly inappropriate and interfere with functioning, at least in certain settings. Ms. P. presented with personality traits that were only somewhat maladaptive; though her behavior was inappropriate, it was unlikely to entirely alienate the directors and producers around whom she felt uncomfortable. In contrast, if an actress compulsively needed to take control in situations that made her anxious, responding to the stresses of auditioning by telling everyone what to do and criticizing and rejecting the direction provided by those running the audition, her behavior would be highly maladaptive—socially far more inappropriate than Ms. P.'s girlish presentation, and more likely to ensure that she did not get the roles she wanted.

Finally, we consider the degree to which personality rigidity is *global*, adversely affecting personality in many or most areas of functioning, versus personality rigidity that is more focal, leading to behaviors that are maladaptive in only a single or a few areas of functioning.

Returning to Ms. P. as a case in point, thus far it appears that her propensity to assume a girlish self-presentation became a significant problem largely in the setting of auditions. Though clearly she had a tendency to hold back and to behave and feel "girlish" as part of her interpersonal style, it appeared that in many settings her behavior was not grossly inappropriate, nor was it significant enough to cause her distress.

Assessment of Personality Types and Higher Level Personality Pathology

After assessing personality organization, making a diagnosis of higher level personality pathology, and completing assessment of severity of personality rigidity, the clinician can consider whether the patient presents with one of the commonly encountered higher level personality disorders or instead presents a mixed picture. This assessment is made predominantly on the basis of the patient's personality traits, complemented by the clinician's response to the patient in the countertransference and his assessment of the patient's core conflicts.

As described in Chapter 2, some patients diagnosed with higher level personality pathology present with one of the "neurotic personality disorders" described in the psychoanalytic literature. The obsessive-compulsive, hysterical, and depressive-masochistic, or depressive, personalities are most commonly described (Kernberg 1984; PDM Task Force 2006). (Obsessive-compulsive and depressive personality disorder are also included in the DSM-IV-TR.) Other patients with higher level personality pathology meet criteria for DSM-IV-TR histrionic, dependent, or avoidant personality disorder. While many patients who meet DSM-IV-TR criteria for these personality disorders have more severe personality pathology, a small, relatively healthy subset of patients in these diagnostic groups have higher level personality pathology. Patients with higher level personality pathology who meet DSM-IV-TR criteria for histrionic, dependent, or avoidant personality disorder typically present with mild identity pathology, manifested as some degree of superficiality or mild instability in the sense of self and/or others in the setting of a capacity to form mutually dependent relationships. Structurally, these patients are best described as having a personality organization that falls in the transitional range between Kernberg's neurotic and borderline levels.

Table 9–4 provides a summary of the higher level personality disorders. For comprehensive discussion of the descriptive, psychodynamic, and clinical features of the higher level personality disorders, we refer the reader to Nancy McWilliams's book *Psychoanalytic Diagnosis: Understanding Personality Structure in the Clinical Process* (1994) and to the *Psychodynamic Diagnostic Manual* published by Alliance of Psychoanalytic Organizations (PDM Task Force 2006).

DIFFERENTIAL TREATMENT PLANNING

The first half of the consultation is organized around acquiring the information needed to make a DSM-IV-TR and structural diagnosis. The second half of the consultation involves 1) sharing the diagnostic impression with the patient, 2) determining treatment goals, 3) reviewing the available treatment options and their relative benefits, and 4) helping the patient make an informed choice with regard to the kind of treatment(s) to pursue.

SHARING THE DIAGNOSTIC IMPRESSION

The second half of the consultation begins with the interviewer sharing his diagnostic impression with the patient. It is important that the consultant review both Axis I symptoms and disorders and personality pathology. The consultant's description of the patient's difficulties and discussion of diagnostic issues should be as clear and specific as possible, and the consultant should avoid using technical terms or jargon. It is our recommendation that when discussing diagnostic issues, the consultant first offer a summary of the patient's symptoms and maladaptive personality traits, inquiring of the patient if the formulation seems accurate and if there is anything the patient would like to add or modify.

In contrast to disorders such as major depression or panic disorder, for which there are clear diagnostic criteria that the consultant can refer to, when it comes to discussing personality pathology with the patient, the consultant has to lean more heavily on his own description and conceptualization of that pathology. When the consultant is discussing higher level personality rigidity with a patient, it is generally not necessary to identify a specific personality type or to use the term "personality disorder," which may be confusing or insulting to patients. Instead, we recommend that the consultant explain the construct of personality rigidity and how it relates to the patient's presenting problems and maladaptive personality traits. For patients who present with

TABLE 9–4. Core features of personality disorders commonly diagnosed in patients with higher level personality pathology

	Introverted ←					→ Extraverted
	Avoidant	Obsessive-compulsive	Depressive	Dependent	Hysterical	Histrionic
Identity	Largely consolidated	Consolidated	Consolidated	Largely consolidated	Consolidated	Largely consolidated
Affective tone	Fearful Depressive	Emotionally constricted	Somber Serious	Anxious	Emotional	Hyperemotional Superficial
Cognitive style	Hypervigilant	Focus on detail	Thoughtful, thorough	Variable	Impressionistic	Superficial
Interpersonal style	Shy Hypersensitive to slights and/or criticism	Controlling and/or sadistic Judgmental	Seeking love Sensitive to loss	Ingratiating Submissive Clinging	Attention seeking Seductive	Demanding of attention Aggressively seductive
Attitude toward self	Inferior Undesirable	Perfectionistic Morally superior	Perfectionistic Self-critical	Ineffectual Needy	Childlike and inadequate, restricted to sexually meaningful settings	Infantile Grandiose Erotized
Common symptoms	Social anxiety Social isolation Imagined derision from others	Anxiety, anxious ruminations	Depression, guilty ruminations	Fears of abandonment Sadness and fear when relationships end	Sexual inhibitions	Sexual promiscuity Affective lability Temper tantrums
Core dynamics	Conflicts around dependency with projection of aggressive self-criticism and wishes to devalue vulnerable objects	Compromise formations around oedipal aggression and dependency with defensive retreat to struggles over control of self and others	Intolerance of aggression, which is turned against the self; conflicts around being cared for as defense against oedipal conflicts	Conflicts around dependency and trust with defensive use of idealization of powerful significant others and devaluation of the self	Oedipal conflicts around sexuality and dependency	Conflicts around dependency with defensive use of sexuality to gratify dependent and aggressive needs

severe personality pathology, discussion will be organized around the construct of identity, helping the patient conceptualize his problems from the perspective of his having an incompletely consolidated or unstable sense of self.

CLINICAL ILLUSTRATION OF SHARING THE DIAGNOSTIC IMPRESSION

As an example of how a consultant might go about sharing his diagnostic impression, let us return to the actress interviewed earlier in this chapter, Ms. P. After interviewing the patient, the consultant might say something along the lines of,

"It sounds to me like you are describing two problems, which may or may not be related. First, you are feeling somewhat depressed, more so than you are accustomed to feeling, and it is not clear what has triggered the change in your mood. I do not think you have a 'clinical' depression that necessarily requires specific treatment. It sounds more like some sort of adjustment reaction, perhaps in response to trying to pursue your dream of acting on stage. Your current difficulties may also have to do with your moving in with your boyfriend. I know you are happy to be living with him and that things are going well. Even so, it is possible that, outside your awareness, there is something about taking this step, about what it means to you to be moving in with him, that is troubling you. So far, does what I'm saying make sense to you?"

If the patient indicates that she is following what the consultant is saying and that it seems plausible to her, he might go on to say something like,

"You have described a second problem, which sounds like it is more chronic than the low mood, having to do with how you view yourself and how you present yourself in certain settings. I suspect this problem is connected to the recent decline in your mood, though it may not be. As I see it, much as you understand that you are a successful and mature performer who is respected by directors and producers, for unclear reasons, when you walk into an audition, you tend to feel like a little girl. These feelings are apparently most acute when you are auditioning for theatre rather than television, and especially when auditioning for men whom you admire and who you suspect are admiring of you as well. Furthermore, this difficulty appears to be part of a more general pattern in which you maintain a girlish image of yourself. Though this does not appear to cause problems in most settings, I suspect when you are anxious this tendency may become more pronounced."

Here, the consultant might pause, again to see if the patient is "with" him. If the patient appears to be following and agreeing, the consultant can continue to share how he thinks about this difficulty:

"I think of the kind of problems you are having in your auditions in terms of what we can call 'rigidity' in your personality. By rigidity, I mean that you can't adjust your behavior in the way you would like to and that would make sense to do. Rather, you keep doing the same thing over and over, despite your best efforts to behave differently. Typically, personality rigidity of this kind is driven by psychological forces that are outside awareness. This is to say that, for reasons you are not aware of, you are automatically and involuntarily driven to feel and to some degree act like a child when you audition. You are driven to do so, even though you understand that this behavior is not appropriate, and even though you would prefer, consciously, to behave differently."

DETERMINING TREATMENT GOALS

Many patients have specific and relatively limited treatment goals, despite their descriptions of broad areas of difficulty during the assessment. For example, we might see a patient with panic attacks, in the context of severe and highly maladaptive personality rigidity, who wants treatment only for his panic attacks; or we might see a patient with global and severe personality rigidity affecting multiple areas of functioning but whose only treatment goal is to deal more effectively with the people he reports to at work.

Conversely, some patients have seemingly infinite and highly unrealistic expectations of what can be accomplished in psychotherapy. For example, we might see a patient who is globally inhibited and self-defeating to a degree that has interfered with her professional, romantic, and social functioning, and who comes to therapy hoping to become outgoing and assertive in all of her interactions, "like my mother." Thus, it is the responsibility of the consultant to help the patient determine exactly what he is seeking treatment for—that is, what he hopes to see ameliorated by the time treatment ends. Further, the consultant should not agree to treatment goals that are simply unrealistic, as, for example, in the case of the patient who would like to change her personality to become more like her mother.

In selecting treatment goals, it is important that the consultant help the patient figure out what his personal goals are—which aspects of his situation are sufficiently troubling to him to warrant treatment. Before establishing treatment goals, the consultant should spend time clarifying in detail the impact of personality rigidity on the patient's functioning. When there are seemingly significant areas of dysfunction that the patient is not manifestly troubled by, the consultant should call this to the patient's attention and explore the implications of the position the patient is taking by not including particular areas of significant maladaptive functioning in the treatment goals.

CLINICAL ILLUSTRATION OF
DETERMINING THE TREATMENT GOALS

As an example of the broad array of treatment goals that a given patient might have, let us return to Ms. P. First, as we have described, the consultant would help Ms. P. formulate the nature of her difficulties. Next, he would help her clarify, among the areas of difficulty described, which are those for which she seeks treatment. For example, it is possible that someone like Ms. P. could present predominantly with concern about her depressed mood. Alternatively, the consultant would want to know whether she had interest in treatment for sexual inhibitions. In the case of Ms. P., the consultant was able to determine a clear and relatively specific treatment goal. Ms. P.'s goal was to modify her need to feel and behave in a girlish fashion in situations in which this behavior was most pronounced and most maladaptive, primarily in auditions and secondarily in her relationship with her fiancé.

DISCUSSING TREATMENT OPTIONS

The nature of the patient's goals determines treatment options. It is the consultant's job to facilitate the patient's making an informed and autonomous decision, guided by the consultant's expertise and recommendations, but ultimately determined by the needs and wishes of the patient, as reflected in his personal goals and level of motivation for treatment. As he reviews treatment options and recommends a particular form of psychotherapy and before beginning treatment, the clinician should initiate a process of obtaining informed consent (Beahrs and Gutheil 2001). It is incumbent upon the clinician to disclose enough information for the patient to make a reasoned decision about whether to undertake the treatment.

Informed decision making begins with the process described above, in which the consultant shares his impressions and diagnostic assessment and then helps the patient clarify his goals. The next step is for the therapist to review possible treatment options, along with potential benefits, costs, and risks of each treatment approach. For example, for a patient with personality rigidity, a brief, supportive, or cognitive-behavioral treatment is less time intensive, less expensive, and perhaps less stressful than DPHP, but will by necessity have less ambitious goals. The elements involved in informed decision making for psychotherapy are outlined in Table 9–5.

For patients with higher level personality pathology who present with complaints related to personality rigidity, treatment options include 1) short-term, focal, psychodynamic psychotherapy; 2) supportive psychotherapy; 3) behavior therapy; 4) cognitive-behavioral treatment; 5) DPHP; and 6) psychoanalysis. If a patient's goal is to modify relatively flexible personality rigidity that is especially troubling or maladaptive in focal areas of functioning, depending upon the patient's specific complaint, a short-term focal, supportive, behavioral, or cognitive behavioral treatment may be sufficient. As personality rigidity becomes more inflexible, less intensive treatments are less likely to be effective, and we believe that DPHP becomes more clearly indicated. Additionally, as personality traits become progressively maladaptive, there is increasing rationale and motivation for intensive treatment.

TABLE 9–5.	Informed consent for dynamic therapy

The goal of the process of informed consent is to facilitate autonomous decision making. Informed consent entails:

- Discussion of the patient's diagnosis and a formulation of the patient's difficulties
- Discussion of the course, etiology, and associated symptoms of the patient's presenting complaints
- Discussion of expected outcome if the patient does not pursue treatment
- Description of DPHP and the associated risks and benefits of DPHP, including the expected duration of treatment and possible side effects (for example, temporary increase in anxiety or other symptoms)
- Discussion of significant alternative treatments with their attendant risks and benefits

Note. DPHP = dynamic psychotherapy for higher level personality pathology.

In cases for which DPHP is indicated, the more focal the area in which personality traits are maladaptive and adversely affect functioning, the more likely DPHP is to be successful. As personality rigidity becomes more global and a cause for severe impairment in many or all areas of functioning, the consultant may consider recommending psychoanalysis. Alternatively, if a patient who presents with global and relatively severe personality rigidity is able to select a specific goal, DPHP is a reasonable treatment recommendation.

It is the role of the consultant to honestly share with the patient his assessment of which treatments will address which aspects of the patient's pathology, as well as the costs, in terms of time, money, and potential side effects of available treatment options. When recommending DPHP, the consultant should describe the potential benefits, as well as the costs and potential risks of the treatment, along with information about the expected course of the patient's personality rigidity without treatment.

To describe DPHP, the consultant might say something like,

"DPHP is a treatment designed to help us learn more about those aspects of your inner experience that underlie the problems that brought you to treatment. Some of the anxiety and concerns driving your behavior may be conscious, while others are likely outside of your conscious awareness. The treatment involves your speaking openly and honestly about what is on your mind while you are in sessions, as this is the most effective way we know of to learn more about your inner life. My role is to help identify the patterns of thinking, behavior, and fantasies that underlie your difficulties. The general idea is that as you better understand the fears and anxieties inside you that are driving your behavior, you will be able to deal with them in a more flexible and adaptive fashion."

In addition, the consultant should explain that DPHP is a twice-weekly treatment that is typically of 1 to 4 years' duration. There are few serious risks associated with the treatment, though the treatment can stir up strong feelings and the patient may experience heightened anxiety or other symptoms as transient "side effects" at various points during the treatment. The patient should understand that, though the consultant recommends DPHP, other treatment options exist, each with its own rationale and risk/benefit profile.

STRUCTURED ASSESSMENT

In a clinical setting, we recommend the clinical interview that we have outlined in this chapter. However, a research setting demands a more structured approach, to ensure that patients are evaluated in a uniform fashion and that diagnostic assessments are reliable across different raters and different sites. To meet these demands and to facilitate the evaluation of personality organization in clinical research trials, we have developed the Structured Interview for Personality Organization (STIPO), which is available on our website (www.borderlinedisorders.com). The semi-structured interview format of the STIPO provides a standardized way to gather information about personality organization and to score it objectively.

Although the STIPO was originally developed for research purposes, we have found that it can serve as a useful educational tool as well. For the clinician who is relatively new to structural assessment and psychodynamic interviewing, the STIPO offers a series of specific questions and follow-up probes that can be used to evaluate the dimensions of personality relevant to assessing the level of personality organization.

Other authors have studied the systematic assessment of patients who present with personality pathology. Piper's object relations interview (see Piper and Duncan 1999) has been used to assess patients, and has been found to predict response to different forms of brief psychotherapy. Westen and Schedler (1999a, 1999b) have developed the Schedler-Westen Assessment Procedure (SWAP), an instrument that uses Q-sort methodology to reliably assess personality and personality pathology. The SWAP is scored on the basis of patients' descriptions of themselves and others, captured in interpersonal narratives in clinical interviews or therapy sessions.

SUGGESTED READINGS

Abraham K: Contributions to the theory of the anal character (1921), in Selected Papers of Karl Abraham, MD. London, Hogarth Press, 1942, pp 370–392
American Psychiatric Association: Resource Document on Principles of Informed Consent in Psychiatry, J Am Acad Psychiatry Law 25:121–125, 1997

Beahrs JO, Gutheil TG: Informed consent in psychotherapy. Am J Psychiatry 158:4–10, 2001

Easser BR, Lesser S: Hysterical personality: a re-evaluation. Psychoanal Q 34:390–405, 1965

Kernberg OF: The structural interview, in Severe Personality Disorders. New Haven, CT, Yale University Press, 1984, pp 27–51

Kernberg OF: Hysterical and histrionic personality disorders, in Aggression in Personality Disorders and Perversions. New Haven, CT, Yale University Press, 1992, pp 52–66

Laughlin HP: The Neuroses. New York, Appleton-Century Crofts, 1967

MacKinnon RA, Michels R, Buckley PJ: The Psychiatric Interview in Clinical Practice, 2nd Edition. Washington, DC, American Psychiatric Publishing, 2006

Westen D, Schedler J: Revising and assessing Axis II, Part I: developing a clinically and empirically valid assessment method. Am J Psychiatry 156:258–272, 1999

Westen D, Schedler J: Revising and assessing Axis II, Part II: toward an empirically based and clinically useful classification of personality disorders. Am J Psychiatry, 156:273–285, 1999

THE PHASES OF TREATMENT

A dynamic psychotherapy can be thought of as having an opening phase, a middle phase, and a termination phase. Although these three phases are not sharply demarcated and gradually flow from one to the next, there are characteristic features of each that can be described and used to conceptualize the flow of treatment. In this chapter we discuss the three phases of dynamic psychotherapy for higher level personality disorder (DPHP) and clinical issues that commonly arise in each of the phases of treatment.

THE OPENING PHASE OF DPHP

The opening phase of DPHP can be as short as several months and as long as a year, depending on the patient's affinity for working in an exploratory treatment and the skill of the therapist. The tasks of the early portions of the opening phase are to explore early resistances to free and open communication, solidify the treatment alliance, explore early character resistances, and identify dominant defensive object relations. By the end of the opening phase, core conflicts and associated object relations will have been identified. As a result of the work of the opening phase, the patient acquires a deepening appreciation of unconscious, dynamic mental processes, along with an increasing capacity for self-observation in areas of conflict.

EXPLORING EARLY RESISTANCE TO
FREE AND OPEN COMMUNICATION

Each patient will respond differently, and characteristically, to the request to communicate openly and freely with the therapist. Some patients find it especially difficult to come to session without a prepared agenda; some others find it difficult to know what to talk about in response to the unstructured request to "say what comes to mind"; and some find it particularly difficult to tolerate silences. The DPHP therapist will pay careful attention to the way the patient responds to the intimate and relatively unstructured nature of the treatment setting. Early interventions will focus on clarifying and exploring anxieties stimulated by the opening phase of treatment, with particular attention to analysis of resistance, focusing on both resistance to free and open communication and character resistances. Exploring the patient's conscious and unconscious resistances to open communication will enable the therapist to identify and describe the object relations being enacted in the treatment.

CLINICAL ILLUSTRATIONS OF EXPLORING EARLY RESISTANCES
TO FREE AND OPEN COMMUNICATION

As an example of an early resistance to free and open communication, consider the patient who, in the early sessions of his treatment, routinely walked into his therapist's office, sat down, and immediately began speaking in a highly detailed way about his day. The patient's tone was extremely earnest, and he continued to speak essentially without a break throughout the hour. In the opening sessions of the treatment, the therapist waited to see if the patient would relax. When the patient's behavior continued unchanged, the therapist decided to intervene.

The therapist interrupted the patient to say that he was getting the impression that the patient was somewhat anxious in his sessions and that one way the patient seemed to be dealing with this anxiety was to come to session and to systematically report recent events, leaving little time for reflection. The patient's initial response to the therapist was that he was trying to give the therapist as much information as possible, in a clear and detailed fashion. After all, the patient asked, wasn't this what the therapist wanted?

It seemed clear that the patient felt criticized. In fact, with further discussion, it turned out that the patient had been carefully pre-selecting material to discuss in each session, virtually rehearsing ahead of time what he would say. As the therapist helped the patient explore his motivation for doing this, it emerged that the patient's behavior was prompted by a concern that if he did not fill the time with information, the therapist would feel displeased by or critical of the patient or think that the patient was not working hard enough or was not "doing it right." Exploration of these anxieties enabled the therapist to describe an object relation of a child-self, fearful of being criticized and manifestly eager to please, in relation to a rigid, demanding, and critical parent, an object relation that was being enacted in the sessions. Making this object relation explicit helped the patient relax and communicate somewhat more spontaneously and comfortably with the therapist. At the same time, exploration of this early transference resistance served as an entry point into exploration of the patient's conflicts in relation to authority figures.

Another patient who had difficulty communicating freely complained that she found it "impossible" to know what to say in session. The silences that ensued were filled with anxiety for the patient. After a time, the therapist suggested that perhaps the patient wished the therapist would be more active and tell her what to talk about, as a way to mitigate her anxiety, and that if so, she must wonder why the therapist was not doing anything to help her when this would be relatively easy.

The patient concurred that these were, indeed, thoughts she had been having. As these early resistances were further explored, it became clear that the unstructured treatment setting, in conjunction with the act of coming for help, had activated an object relation of a needy child-self in relation to a withholding and selfish maternal figure. As in the preceding example, as this object relation, now activated in the transference, was identified and explored, the patient felt less paralyzed in session and was able to associate and communicate more freely. In this process, therapist and patient began to link this object relation to recurrent difficulties the patient faced in her intimate life.

SOLIDIFYING THE THERAPEUTIC ALLIANCE

Patients with higher level personality pathology bring to treatment a well-developed capacity to form a therapeutic alliance with a concerned and helpful professional[1] (Bender 2005; Gibbons et al. 2003; Piper et al. 1991). Thus, in DPHP, the treatment alliance is typically established easily and naturally in the early contacts between therapist and patient. Furthermore, analysis of early resistances to free and open communication will fortify the developing alliance as the patient joins with the therapist to explore the patient's early responses to the treatment setting.

There is, however, a group of patients with higher level personality pathology who do have some degree of difficulty in solidifying a treatment alliance. For these patients, the treatment setting quickly and relatively intensely activates highly maladaptive defensive object relations that powerfully color the patient's experience of the therapeutic relationship in the opening phase of the treatment. Ultimately, this kind of distortion of the therapeutic relationship becomes the basis for transference analysis. How-

---

[1]This is very much in contrast to the situation encountered with patients with more severe personality pathology, where the early treatment alliance is typically unstable and often is built on idealization of the therapist.

ever, for patients with greater personality rigidity whose conflicts are immediately triggered by the treatment situation, early and relatively powerful negative transferences will distort the relationship with the therapist more quickly and more intensely than is typically seen with patients with higher level personality pathology. These early transference reactions can interfere with the natural development of a therapeutic alliance.

The DPHP therapist deals with this development by actively identifying and exploring these transferences. This process will help promote the treatment alliance by facilitating the patient's ability to observe and thereby to distance himself, to some degree, from negative transferences that color the treatment relationship. In essence, analysis of early negative transferences helps the patient more clearly distinguish between the helping therapist in his professional role and the negative transference object.

CLINICAL ILLUSTRATION OF EXPLORING DIFFICULTY IN ESTABLISHING A THERAPEUTIC ALLIANCE

As an example of a patient who had a relatively difficult time establishing a therapeutic alliance, consider the patient who, from the earliest phases of consultation, was constantly correcting the therapist and getting into power struggles over whether the therapist had accurately understood what the patient had told him about himself. It appeared that the patient had little faith in the therapist's ability to understand him, let alone help him, and feared that he was putting himself in the hands of an incompetent doctor.

The therapist did not feel that a therapeutic alliance was developing. In the countertransference, the therapist felt critically attacked and devalued by the patient. He wondered if the patient would drop out of treatment. The patient had initially come to treatment complaining of difficulty getting along with his boss, whom the patient found critical and devaluing, as well as with his subordinates, whom the patient found incompetent. In his own mind, the therapist was able to describe the object relation that was being enacted: one party in a dominant position was critical and devaluing, while the other, in a subordinate position, felt incompetent and fearful of being rejected. The therapist noted how he himself was moving from feeling criticized and incompetent to feeling devaluing and rejecting of the patient. The therapist inferred that the patient's unpleasant behavior in part might be motivated by the patient's fears of being devalued and criticized by the therapist and perhaps, ultimately, rejected by him.

Over the ensuing sessions, the therapist shared with the patient his understanding of the object relation being enacted and linked it to the patient's difficulties with both his boss and his employees. The therapist did this from a position of technical neutrality, clearly communicating concern for the patient while retaining a respectful, noncritical, and not-devaluing attitude in response to the patient's initial rebuffs. The therapist described the patient's critical and devaluing attitude and his apparent concern that the therapist was incompetent and had nothing to offer the patient.

The therapist also pointed out to the patient that he had come to the therapist for help. If the patient really felt that the therapist could not possibly understand him, the patient would do better to choose another therapist. However, if the patient felt the therapist might have something to offer, it would make sense to try to understand why the patient treated the therapist in the way that he did and to explore how this might relate to the problems that had brought him to treatment.

As the therapist maintained an attitude of curiosity and concern, neither devaluing nor criticizing the patient, the patient started to reflect on the therapist's comments, acknowledging that the therapist made a valid point and considering that perhaps the therapist *did* know what he was doing. As this early character resistance was worked through, patient and therapist developed a sense of working together to understand the forces in the patient that could interfere with the treatment and interfere with the patient's feeling helped by the therapist.

The opening phase of treatment is typically longer with patients who have more difficulty solidifying an alliance. With these patients, time must be devoted in the early phases of treatment to identifying, and to some degree working through, the initial resistances that interfere with establishing an alliance between the patient's observing self and the therapist in role. In contrast, for patients who form an alliance more naturally, the opening phase passes more quickly and smoothly because the patient is quickly able to collaborate with the therapist to identify and explore his anxieties about and resistances to immersing himself in the treatment and the therapeutic relationship.

POSITIVE TRANSFERENCE

We have illustrated how early negative transferences can interfere with solidification of the therapeutic alliance in the opening phase of DPHP. In contrast, early positive transferences promote and support the developing alliance. As a result, in DPHP, we typically do not explore or analyze what are often referred to as "benign positive transferences"—relatively nonconflictual transferences to the helping therapist. Rather than analyzing these transferences, in DPHP we use them as a vehicle to promote the alliance and to facilitate exploration of the patient's conflictual object relations.

Benign positive transferences are to be distinguished from seemingly positive transferences that are being used defensively. The DPHP therapist can make this distinction by keeping in mind that defensively mobilized positive transferences—which defend against activation of conflictual dependent, aggressive, and erotic object relations—tend to be more highly affectively charged, less well integrated, and more idealizing than do benign positive transferences, which have a more neutral quality. In DPHP, idealizing transferences are analyzed by using the standard approach to the analysis of defensive object relations.

EXPLORATION OF EARLY CHARACTER RESISTANCES

We described the central role of the analysis of resistance in the technique of DPHP in Chapter 7 ("The Techniques of DPHP, Part 2: Intervening"). If we define resistance as activation of the patient's defensive operations in the treatment, and in particular in the transference, then it follows that we will routinely see enactment of the patient's character defenses in his interpersonal interactions with the therapist, especially in the opening phase of the treatment.

The examples provided earlier in this chapter—the earnest patient who always came prepared and the argumentative patient who was always dismissive and critical—both illustrate how patients can quickly activate and enact their character defenses in relation to the therapist. Both these patients were doing in the session what they habitually did outside the session. Enactment of the patient's character defenses in the opening phase of treatment enables the DPHP therapist to describe and explore the object relations embedded in the patient's maladaptive character traits and ultimately to identify the conflicts underlying the patient's chief complaints.

In sum, in the early phases of DPHP we identify the patient's recurrent, maladaptive ways of facing the world and interacting with others as they are enacted both within the treatment and outside it. This makes it possible to describe the object relations embedded in these behaviors and to explore how their automatic and habitual enactment functions to ward off underlying core conflicts. Analysis of the dominant defensive object relations paves the way for identifying the patient's core conflicts and for using the strategies, techniques, and tactics that we described in Part II of this volume to analyze the conflicts underlying the patient's presenting complaints.

MARKERS OF CHANGE AND TRANSITION TO THE MIDDLE PHASE

Patients with higher level personality pathology typically come to treatment with a fairly well developed capacity for self-observation. However, in areas of conflict, self-observation is typically more limited, hampered by the patient's defensive operations. In the opening phase of DPHP, patients develop a greater capacity to introspect and to observe their own thoughts, feelings, and behaviors in areas of conflict. This shift can be understood in terms of fortification of the patient's capacity for self-observation and introspection as a result of the therapist's exploration of the patient's inner life from a position of technical neutrality. The increase in capacity for self-observation and introspection seen in the opening phase of DPHP is typically accompanied by an enhanced awareness of fantasy and other transient thoughts and feelings that the patient would have disregarded or not consciously registered in the past because they are related to conflict.

During the opening phase, patients become familiar with the idea of "unconscious motivation." This development follows upon the therapist's tactful and systematic exploration of the patient's defensive operations and underlying anxieties. Patients come to appreciate that many of the maladaptive behavior traits and repetitive thoughts, feelings, and emotional experiences that brought them to treatment are both motivated and meaningful, and they come to question familiar rationalizations about their personality traits and maladaptive behaviors, which become more ego dystonic.

As patients move through the opening phase, they begin to develop the capacity to tolerate awareness of previously dissociated and repressed aspects of their inner lives and to reflect upon conflictual experiences of self and others. The emergence of repressed and dissociated mental representations into consciousness is facilitated by the therapist's interventions—specifically clarification, confrontation, and analysis of resistance from a position of technical neutrality. The patient's capacity to tolerate awareness of conflictual object relations is supported by the tolerant and accepting attitude of the therapist. The emergence of an enhanced capacity to tolerate awareness of conflictual object relations is an early sign of decreasing personality rigidity and is one of the markers of transition to the middle phase. This capacity may be accompanied by an increased capacity to work in the transference.

THE MIDDLE PHASE OF DPHP

The middle phase of DPHP can last anywhere from 1 to 3 years. The dominant tasks of the middle phase correspond to the strategies of treatment described in Chapter 5 ("The Strategies of DPHP and the Treatment Setting"). Because most of this handbook is devoted to describing these strategies and how to implement them, we comment here only briefly on the central tasks of the middle phase, emphasizing typical clinical developments seen in that phase.

EXPLORATION AND WORKING THROUGH OF OBJECT RELATIONS DEFINING CORE CONFLICTS

As a result of the work of the opening phase of treatment, the patient entering the middle phase has an appreciation of the nature of his core conflicts. Defensive object relations have been explored, and conflictual object relations corresponding to the unconscious motivations, anxieties, and fantasies underlying the difficulties that brought the patient to treatment have been identified. The central task of the middle phase is to *work through* core conflicts as conflictual object relations are enacted in the treatment and in the patient's daily interactions with others.

The term *working through* refers to the repeated enactment, identification, and exploration of a particular constellation of conflictual object relations, over time and in a variety of contexts. The process of working through begins in the middle phase of treatment, continues into the termination phase, and is completed by the patient, working independently of the therapist, after termination. However, the bulk of working through takes place in the middle phase of DPHP. In sum, the central tasks of the middle phase of DPHP are to explore and work through the conflictual object relations and associated anxieties underlying the patient's presenting complaints so that they can be more flexibly integrated into the patient's subjective experience. It is the process of working through core conflicts in relation to the treatment goals that leads to reduction in personality rigidity and to symptomatic improvement.

CAPACITY TO TOLERATE MORE "PRIMITIVE" MENTAL CONTENTS AND AFFECTS

The object relations that emerge early in DPHP are predominantly defensive and are relatively accessible to consciousness and relatively well integrated. Furthermore, when underlying conflictual motivations and associated anxieties are represented early in treatment, it is in a relatively "sanitized" or "civilized" form. These representations are most accurately described as derivatives of the underlying conflict and generally do not take the form of direct expressions or representations of underlying conflictual motivations and anxieties. In contrast, as the patient moves into and through the middle phase, the object relations uncovered more directly represent conflictual motivations and associated anxieties.

During the middle phase of DPHP the patient gains greater access to his inner life and becomes more tolerant of awareness of unacceptable, warded-off parts of his inner world. As a result, the object relations mobilized during this middle portion of the treatment may be more polarized, more one-dimensional, and less well differentiated (referring to the content and the quality of representation of internal object relations that are enacted) and more concrete and affectively charged (referring to the quality of experience associated with the internal object relations that are enacted) than those seen earlier. The patient's capacity to tolerate awareness of a broader range of psychological experience is supported by the tolerant and accepting attitude of the containing therapist, as threatening, conflictual object relations are enacted in the treatment and put into words.

The process wherein the patient in DPHP is increasingly able to tolerate awareness of previously repressed, unacceptable, and often highly charged aspects of his inner life is sometimes referred to as "therapeutic regression" or "deepening" of the treatment. The object relations that now become conscious and are enacted in the treatment are less well integrated, or more "primitive," than is typical of the conscious experience of the individual with higher level personality pathology. Paradoxically, this "regressive" shift toward more poorly integrated object relations and affects signifies progression of the treatment in the middle phase, as the patient gains access to previously inaccessible mental contents. Therapeutic regression and deepening of the treatment are the hallmarks of the middle phase of DPHP.

INTENSIFICATION OF TRANSFERENCE AND INCREASING FOCUS ON WORKING IN THE TRANSFERENCE

Some patients with higher level personality pathology have a great affinity for working in the transference, whereas other patients do not easily develop or make use of transferential feelings. However, although timing may vary, most patients develop an increasing capacity to make use of the transference as they progress through the middle phase of treatment.

This facility reflects the increased capacity to tolerate awareness of conflictual motivations and representations; patients work more effectively and comfortably with transferential material as they become less afraid of experiencing conflictual aggressive, dependent, and erotic wishes, needs, and fears. As the patient in DPHP moves through the middle phase and the treatment deepens, previously repressed conflictual object relations become accessible to consciousness, and they are often enacted in the transference. The object relations enacted in the transference in the middle phase of DPHP tend to be more highly affectively charged than the transferences activated earlier in the treatment.

FURTHER COMMENTS ON WORKING THROUGH OF OBJECT RELATIONS DEFINING CORE CONFLICTS: PARANOID ANXIETIES BEFORE DEPRESSIVE ANXIETIES

The topic of the various phases of treatment raises the question of whether there is a particular order in which we typically explore the patient's conflicts in DPHP. First, it needs to be said that there is tremendous variation with regard to the order in which conflicts unfold in treatment, varying from patient to patient and depending upon which conflicts are most threatening to a given patient. Second, we have already described how, when it comes to deciding when to intervene, the rules of affective dominance and working from surface to depth will guide the therapist's interventions.

However, in the middle phase, when the patient's core conflicts have been identified and explored and are being worked through in relation to presenting complaints, the therapist will often find himself faced within a given session with two sets of anxieties, both being enacted in the treatment and both conscious. Enactment of one set of anxieties defends against activation of the other, and vice versa. In this situation, it falls to the therapist to decide which set of anxieties to view as primary at any given moment and which to see as defensive.

When confronted with enactment of two different sets of anxieties, one used to defend against the other, it is generally preferable to work through paranoid anxieties before addressing depressive anxieties. As discussed in Chapter 3, a *paranoid orientation* implies that threatening aspects of the patient's internal world are split off from self experience and projected into an object. As a result, the patient feels himself to be in danger in relation to an object perceived as in some way threatening. Responsibility and guilt are located externally, and the dominant affect is fear. In contrast, a *depressive orientation* implies the capacity to contain conflictual motivations and emotional states rather than project them. Here the patient fears not for himself but for his objects, who are in danger as a result of the patient's own aggressive and self-serving motivations. The dominant affects associated with depressive anxiety are guilt and loss, often in conjunction with a wish to make reparation.

Paranoid anxieties are associated with relatively polarized or one-dimensional, all-good or all-bad images of self and other. This is to say that, if I have a paranoid orientation, the person whom I fear and loathe is entirely separate from the person whom I love and trust; if I feel hateful or competitive, it is because the object of my hostility is entirely worthy of being hated or defeated. (Note that there is no conflict as long as I maintain separation between the two—loving and hateful—sets of object relations.) Depressive anxieties, on the other hand, are associated with relatively well-integrated, or ambivalent, experiences of self and other; the person toward whom I am potentially destructive is also someone I love and trust; I am a person who is both loving and destructive, as is my object. (Note that conflict is inevitable in this setting.)

Working through paranoid anxieties and moving toward a more predominantly depressive orientation enhances the patient's capacity to sustain an increasingly deep, stable, and complex image of himself and his objects. Because guilt and mourning are most fully experienced in relation to whole, ambivalent objects (Klein 1935; Steiner 1993), addressing paranoid anxieties before depressive anxieties in therapy facilitates the working through of depressive anxieties. In contrast, if depressive anxieties are addressed before paranoid anxieties are explored, there is a risk of paranoid anxieties simply "going underground." In this situation, paranoid conflicts may become relatively inaccessible to exploration while at the same time interfering with the complete working through of depressive anxieties.

The rule of addressing paranoid before depressive anxieties applies to both the micro process within a given session and to the macro process over months and even years of treatment. On a macro level, as paranoid anxieties are worked through during the middle phase, depressive anxieties gradually become more consistently the focus of treatment. On a micro level, once the patient's core paranoid and depressive anxieties and the associated object relations have been identified and explored in treatment, the patient will tend to oscillate between paranoid and depressive dynamics as part of the process of working through. Thus although the overall trajectory of the treatment is to more solidly establish a depressive level of functioning in areas of conflict, during the course of treatment from moment to moment and session to session patients will typically oscillate between depressive and paranoid orientations.

CLINICAL ILLUSTRATION OF EXPLORING PARANOID ANXIETIES BEFORE DEPRESSIVE ANXIETIES

A 25-year-old law school student presented after failing the bar exam. During the opening months of treatment, she assumed an attitude toward the therapist that was both childlike and excessively ingratiating. This object relation was explored and understood initially in terms of the patient's fears of a maternal figure who was competitive with and potentially undermining of the patient. As these anxieties were partially worked through, the patient became aware of the degree to which she herself felt competitive with both her mother and her roommate. The patient unhappily acknowledged that at some level, she derived pleasure from knowing that mother had always wanted and never had a profession, whereas the patient was hoping for a career, and that similarly, her roommate was unhappily without a partner, whereas the patient was happily involved with a new man.

Nine months into the therapy, the patient accepted a proposal of marriage from the man she had been dating. In the ensuing weeks, the therapist noted that the patient was increasingly deferential in relation to the therapist in a fashion reminiscent of her behavior during the opening months of treatment. The therapist pointed this out to the patient, who acknowledged having been aware of wishes to please and to elevate the therapist in relation to herself. She suspected it had something to do with her recent engagement and in some way with her mother.

As the therapist listened to the patient, she considered how to intervene. She could focus on defenses against depressive anxieties and guilt by linking the patient's submissive behavior to efforts not to look or to feel too fortunate, for fear of leaving those less fortunate—her mother, her roommate, and perhaps the therapist as well—feeling bad. On the other hand, the therapist could focus on defenses against paranoid anxieties, linking the patient's submissive behavior to efforts to ward off a retaliatory attack from an essentially "bad" maternal figure who would resent the patient's happiness and success. Both sets of dynamics were clearly active and had already been explored. Both sets of conflicts were affectively charged and relatively accessible to consciousness.

Following the principle of addressing paranoid anxieties before depressive, the therapist opted to begin by addressing the patient's concerns about being attacked by her mother and somehow resented by the therapist. The therapist's rationale was that exploring and further working through the paranoid version of the patient's competitive struggle with a maternal figure would help her better contain her own competitive and hostile wishes and would at the same time facilitate her maintaining a better-integrated, ambivalent view of her mother, one that acknowledged the mother's vulnerability in the face of the patient's aggression. The capacity to better hold onto an ambivalent image of her relationship with her mother would, in turn, facilitate the patient's working through of depressive anxieties at a deeper level than would be possible if the therapist were to skip over paranoid concerns and immediately address defenses against depressive anxieties.

DEPRESSIVE ANXIETIES DEFEND AGAINST PARANOID: THE "MORAL DEFENSE"

We have already discussed how, in the patient with higher level personality pathology, a paranoid orientation can be activated at both the micro and macro levels to defend against depressive anxieties. At this point, we would like to comment on a particular type of character defense in which depressive object relations and anxieties are enacted to defend against the activation of paranoid object relations on the one hand and against the loss of an idealized caretaking relationship on the other. This defensive operation was first described by Ronald Fairbairn (1943), a Scottish analyst, who referred to this phenomenon as the "moral defense" or the "defense of the superego." Fairbairn was, in essence, making the observation that, sometimes, prominent and conscious feelings of guilt, loss, inferiority, self-criticism, and "badness" do not reflect depressive anxieties in relation to oedipal or depressive conflicts but rather can be best understood as defensive object relations that support repression of paranoid anxieties associated with dependent object relations.

Fairbairn's theory of the moral defense emerged from observing children who had been abused by caretakers. Fairbairn noted that, more often than not, rather than blaming their caretakers for being abusive, these children tended to idealize their caretakers while seeing themselves as "bad." On the one hand, this psychological situation translates into the conscious experience on the part of the child that the abuse is "my fault" and therefore somehow "under my control." On the other hand, this conscious depressive experience of self and other functions to support repression of paranoid anxieties associated with being dependent on callous, unavailable, chaotic, cruel, or exploitive caretakers. In essence, the child's experience is that "I am somehow bad or inadequate, which explains why I am treated poorly by a caretaker who is not bad."

Fairbairn's elaboration of this understanding is that the child is highly motivated to see his parents as essentially good, which is analogous, psychologically, to living in a world in which goodness and sanity prevail. By assuming that he is at fault, then, the child can create or protect an idealized caretaking relationship while successfully repressing the paranoid aspects of that relationship. This psychological situation provides the child with a fantasy of control. Rather than feeling that "I am a helpless victim of people who should love and take care of me but apparently do not," the child prefers to feel that "I am a bad child deserving of mistreatment, but if, someday, I can get it right, I will be loved."

Although the idea of the moral defense emerged from observations of children who had been abused, this constellation of defenses can be found in a broad array of patients who protect themselves from awareness of parental indifference or hostility. In patients with higher level personality pathology, the moral defense often presents in the form of feelings of depression and problems with self-esteem, reflecting the predominance of conscious, defensive object relations organized around a view of the self as unlovable or rightfully unloved. Typically, these self representations are grossly discordant with how others feel about the patient as well as with how the therapist experiences the patient in the countertransference. In essence, these patients are generally caring, giving, and decent people who appear to be totally mired down and invested in hating themselves, not as an expression of unconscious guilt but rather as a highly motivated effort to sustain an image of a sane and caring world of good objects that is free of paranoid anxieties.

If we consider the moral defense from the perspective of the model of unconscious conflict outlined in this manual, we can describe how defensive, self-blaming object relations support repression of paranoid anxieties while maintaining the belief in an idealized caretaking relationship. The underlying conflictual motivation here is the wish to be a loving and gratified child who is the focus of attention for a loving caretaker. Patients who rely on the moral defense cannot tolerate consciously experiencing enactment of this highly pleasurable and longed-for dependent object relation. As such a patient begins to experience himself as a deserving recipient of loving care, activation of paranoid anxieties occurs ("my caretaker hates and abuses me") and painful feelings of loss ensue ("my caretaker could never love me as I wish to be loved"), feelings that are otherwise unconscious.

These painful affects motivate intensification of defensive object relations as the patient resorts to vehemently insisting on his own "badness."
To the degree that this defense fails to support repression of paranoid anxieties, the patient will consciously experience malignant representations of
caretaking relationships associated with feelings of fear and hostility and,
ultimately, painful feelings of loss.

What we see clinically is that, as the patient's defensive experience is
challenged—either in life, on occasions when he must acknowledge that he
is truly loved, or in treatment, when his self-flagellation is confronted as defensive—he responds by becoming even more self-critical in an effort to
support repression of paranoid object relations that threaten to emerge into
consciousness as soon as he starts to question his "badness" or unworthiness. When defensive efforts ultimately fail, the patient may have frankly
paranoid thoughts and feelings as underlying, paranoid-dependent object
relations emerge into consciousness and are enacted in the patient's current
interpersonal relationships. Working through the moral defense thus entails the patient's tolerance of awareness of these paranoid object relations
and, ultimately, the working through of identifications with both sides of
this object relation in conjunction with mourning the loss of highly valued,
idealized images of relationships with caretakers.

The technical approach taken in DPHP when depressive anxieties support repression of paranoid, dependent object relations is no different from
the approach we have outlined for analyzing more straightforward depressive and paranoid conflicts. However, this is a clinical situation in which it
is especially important that the therapist not let theory lead him but instead
keep an open mind to what the patient is communicating.

It can be tempting, for example, for the therapist to immediately assume
that the patient's self-criticism reflects unconscious guilt. In the setting of
the moral defense, however, suggesting that unconscious guilt is the root
cause of the patient's self-criticism can lead the therapist to make inaccurate
interpretations. Interpretations aimed at identifying unconscious guilt will
support repression of underlying paranoid object relations rather than allow such object relations to emerge into consciousness, where they can provide the patient opportunity to work through anxieties associated with the
wish to feel like a beloved and loving child.

CLINICAL ILLUSTRATION OF THE MORAL DEFENSE

A 50-year-old homemaker, married and the mother of grown children, presented to treatment after having been unexpectedly and inexplicably attacked
and rejected by her best friend of many years. The patient came to treatment
depressed. She described how the episode had reinforced a lifelong view of

herself as "dispensable" and that, regardless of what her husband told her, she could not get past feeling that somehow she had been at fault.

This patient had devoted most of her adult life to caring for others: her children, husband, elderly parents, a chronically ill sibling, various other relatives, and an extended circle of friends. Yet, she explained to the therapist, she felt herself to be "of no value" and believed that she could "disappear and no one would notice." The patient came to treatment only because her husband insisted that she get help. The husband also insisted on attending the initial visit, anticipating that the patient would present herself in a sufficiently devalued light so as to make it difficult for the therapist to appreciate the highly unrealistic and defensive nature of her devalued and self-critical view of herself.

The transference during the opening months of the treatment was characterized by enactment of an object relation of a "dispensable" little girl, grateful for any care and attention she might receive from a maternal figure who was idealized as giving, knowing, and "important" yet who was at the same time unconcerned about the little girl's needs. During this period, the therapist pointed out the patient's investment in maintaining this view of things—for example, by always minimizing her own successes and importance to others while failing to notice or acknowledge the potential failings or limitations of others, including the therapist. The therapist also pointed out that whenever there was a chink in this defensively armored view of the world, the patient became anxious and self-critical.

Six months into the treatment, the patient was selected to receive an award in recognition of her service to a national organization, and she was at the same time offered a highly influential, salaried administrative position in the same organization. The patient's initial response was to feel "flattered" and "unworthy," and she assumed she would turn down the offer. Her husband, however, insisted that she was by far the best qualified person for the job, and he would hear nothing of her turning it down. The patient then considered accepting the position.

For the first time in her life, she began to feel quite paranoid. She described to her therapist the feeling that her husband wanted her to take the job only because of the money she would earn. All of a sudden, she saw him as an "exploiter" rather than as a "protector." Similarly, the patient felt that the therapist had no genuine interest in helping her but was actually thinking about his own personal matters as she spoke to him. Although at times the patient had a sense that she was being unreasonable, these thoughts about both her husband and her therapist were highly affectively charged and seemed credible to the patient. This relatively intense reaction came and went over the course of several days before dissipating.

The patient and her therapist spent the next several months analyzing and working through the conflict that had been activated by the patient's successes and the feeling of being admired and loved. It emerged that, during her "reaction," the patient's subjective experience had been flooded by a paranoid object relation of a selfish, callous, and exploitive maternal figure upon whom the patient was dependent. Enactment of this object relation was associated with feelings of hostility, fear, and frank paranoia. These paranoid object relations that had finally broken through the patient's very rigid depressive defenses had, until now, been entirely unconscious.

As this object relation was identified, explored, and worked through, it was linked to the patient's relationship with a mother who had been preoccupied with the patient's chronically ill sibling. The patient had always idealized the mother as "a saint" and had consciously assumed that she had had a happy childhood in the care of a mother who had given her everything that she had a right to reasonably ask for. However, over time, deeply buried feelings of having been neglected and at times treated cruelly by her mother began to emerge, and it seemed that the problems between the two of them went far beyond her mother's having been preoccupied with the patient's chronically ill sister, to the neglect of the patient.

During the ensuing months, the patient came to accept that in retrospect, her mother's behavior throughout her childhood and much of her adulthood had frequently been visibly hostile. In fact, it emerged that relatives and friends had commented on it over the years, but the patient had neither registered her mother's attitude nor taken in the comments of those around her. She came to understand that her mother's hostility and resentment, and her own reciprocal resentment and hostility toward her mother, were psychological realities that she had not been able to tolerate and had instead split off and repressed. Repression of paranoid object relations had been supported by clinging to the defensive object relation of a good mother with a dispensable child, thus allowing the continued hope of an idealized caretaking relationship.

When patients of this kind are treated in DPHP, much of the process of working through involves tolerating and mourning the loss of idealized images of dependent relations. This process will be accompanied by an increased capacity on the part of the patient to realistically experience and tolerate aggression and resentment, whether directed toward or stemming from people whom the patient loves and depends on. In the end, the patient will be left with a newfound sense of deserving love and care.

Even though activation and enactment of paranoid object relations can be dramatic, and working through paranoid anxieties can be challenging and time consuming, the central anxiety that this group of patients struggles with is the painful loss of an ideal, caring mother or other caregiver in relation to an ideal self who is free of aggression and entirely worthy of love and care.

NEGATIVE THERAPEUTIC REACTION

The term *negative therapeutic reaction* describes a situation in which a patient makes a therapeutic gain and then reacts by becoming more symptomatic, anxious, or depressed or by undoing the gains made (Sandler et al. 1992). Although negative therapeutic reactions can occur in any phase of treatment, they are most common in the middle phase of treatment of higher level personality pathology, as the patient begins to develop a realistic sense of the help provided by the therapist and the treatment.

In patients with higher level personality pathology, the dynamics of the negative therapeutic reaction often have to do with the patient's guilt, either conscious or unconscious, about receiving help or making gains. It is common for patients to feel undeserving of the therapist's help or to worry that any gains made will in some way take place at the expense of others or will "leave behind" people whom the patient cares about. Negative therapeutic reactions of this kind, which reflect depressive anxieties, need to be painstakingly worked through—for some patients, many times—over the course of the middle phase and will be reworked during termination.

Negative therapeutic reactions are not always the result of depressive conflicts, and it is important to keep in mind that sometimes, negative therapeutic reactions reflect defenses against paranoid anxieties. In this context, the patient's recognition that the therapist has been helpful or that the therapist has something meaningful to offer may make the therapist seem "too powerful" in the patient's eyes. As a result, the therapist's help can stimulate feelings of inferiority, envy, or hostility as well as fears of being exploited or controlled, accompanied by impulses to undo whatever gains have been made. Negative therapeutic reactions as a result of paranoid anxieties associated with envy are common in patients with severe personality disorders and in narcissistic patients in particular. Although less common, this form of negative therapeutic reaction can also be seen in patients with higher level personality pathology. Patients with higher level personality pathology and prominent narcissistic conflicts are especially prone to negative therapeutic reactions as a result of envy.

CLINICAL ILLUSTRATION OF
NEGATIVE THERAPEUTIC REACTIONS

To illustrate the two forms of negative therapeutic reaction and how they can present in DPHP, let us return to the patient described earlier in this chapter who was so difficult and argumentative in the opening phase of his treatment, enacting the object relation of a critical and devaluing superior and an incompetent subordinate. In the early portion of the middle phase of this patient's treatment, he was told in his performance review at work that he was doing a better job as a manager. The patient felt pleased, but he came into his session that evening wondering if things might be going too slowly in the treatment and whether a different therapist or a different kind of treatment might be more efficient. The patient complained that he had been feeling down. As the session progressed, he began to feel a bit paranoid about the therapist; he wondered why the therapist had not raised the possibility of a change in the treatment and also why the therapist did not respond directly to the patient's comments about making a change.

In response, the therapist pointed out the apparent contradiction between the patient's current attitude toward the therapist and the treatment, on the one hand, and his positive evaluation at work, on the other. It seemed that the treatment was helping the patient with the difficulties for which he had come for help, yet at exactly this moment the patient found himself especially dissatisfied. The therapist went on to suggest that perhaps, and paradoxically so, the patient was not entirely happy to find that the therapist had been *able* to help. When the patient indicated that he did not disagree, the therapist went on to suggest that perhaps the situation left the patient feeling that the therapist was "too powerful." It was almost as though the therapist's help left the patient feeling diminished, as though the therapist were "showing him up" by being able to help him with something he had not been able to do on his own.

The therapist also raised the possibility that recent gains made in the treatment not only left the patient feeling down about himself but also suspicious of the therapist. After all, if the therapist had "goods" to offer, why had he not shared them more efficiently? The patient acknowledged that he had, in passing, had this thought; furthermore, when he considered it, he realized that he *had* been feeling mistrustful of the therapist that day.

Later in the middle phase of the treatment, the patient again received a positive performance review at work. The previous 6 months of his treatment had been devoted to understanding and working through his conflicted feelings about his boss. In the patient's review, the boss commented on how much he had been enjoying working with the patient. The boss went on to say that he had highly recommended the patient for a promotion.

The next day, the patient came into session to share the good news but also to say that he was suddenly feeling depressed—at least as depressed as he had on first coming to treatment. He wondered once again if the treatment was really helping, and toward the end of the session he announced that he had decided to end the treatment. After all, it might be that he had accomplished all he could.

Once again, the therapist linked the patient's current depressed mood and nihilistic attitude toward his treatment to favorable developments at work. The therapist suggested that perhaps the patient was now feeling depressed and wanting to end his treatment because, out of his awareness, he felt guilty about or undeserving of the help he was receiving in therapy. The patient immediately commented that he had been able to enjoy his boss's encouraging words for only a minute, and then he had started to worry that the promotion would put him in the position of competing with his boss—and also, perhaps, of earning more money than the therapist would ever be able to earn.

WORKING THROUGH OF DEVELOPMENTAL ANTECEDENTS OF CONFLICTUAL OBJECT RELATIONS

In Chapter 7 ("The Techniques of DPHP, Part 2: Intervening"), in introducing the process of interpretation, we commented that in DPHP we do not emphasize "genetic" interpretations that link current conflicts to the patient's early history but instead generally focus on conflictual object relations as they are enacted in the here and now, both in the patient's current life and in the treatment. However, as a patient moves through the middle phase and core conflicts are worked through, it can be helpful to link the object relations that are being worked through in the here and now to important figures and experiences from the patient's developmental history. Where premature interpretation of the role of the past generally leads to intellectualized discussions with limited therapeutic benefit, well-timed interpretations that link the patient's early history to object relations that are alive in the treatment can provide additional depth and meaning to the process of working through.

Thus, in the middle phase of DPHP, identifying and exploring the links between the object relations that define the patient's core conflicts and important figures and events in his developmental history becomes a part of the process of working through.

MARKERS OF CHANGE AND TRANSITION
TO THE TERMINATION PHASE

Whereas in the early portions of the middle phase it may take several sessions to identify and fully explore a given conflict and the associated object relations, by the end of the middle phase we often see enactment and analysis of an entire conflict, defense, anxiety, and conflictual motivation, or even of several core conflicts, within a single session. This shift reflects both decreasing personality rigidity on the part of the patient, so that the various components of a conflict are readily accessible to consciousness, and the familiarity of both patient and therapist with the dominant defensive and impulsive object relations associated with the patient's core conflicts, so that they can be relatively quickly and easily identified. In addition, we typically see an increase in the patient's capacity to independently observe, reflect upon, and work through conflicts that are being enacted, often with little need for the therapist to intervene, as the patient moves through the latter portion of the middle phase and toward termination.

In the middle phase of treatment, object relations associated with conflicts underlying the patient's presenting complaints are repeatedly enacted and worked through. As a result of this process, conflictual object relations gradually become better integrated and less threatening, and they assume a more ambivalent and overall positive coloring. Thus, whereas in the early and middle portions of the middle phase of DPHP emergence of more poorly integrated object relations is an indication of progression of the treatment, by the end of the middle phase progress is marked by the gradual integration of representations and affects associated with conflictual object relations. These better-integrated object relations are consciously tolerated by the patient and acknowledged as conflictual aspects of his self experience. This process heralds the transition from the middle to the termination phase.

THE TERMINATION PHASE

The termination phase is typically of 3 to 6 months' duration and begins when patient and therapist decide to end the treatment. The goal of the termination phase is to consolidate the gains made during treatment and to work through the anxieties activated by the prospect of ending. During the course of treatment, noting gains and making progress toward attaining the treatment goals prepares the patient for termination by helping him maintain awareness that treatment will indeed end and that the goals of the treatment are finite. The manner in which separations, losses, disappointments, and successes have been dealt with during the course of treatment, along with information gathered about the nature of the patient's conflicts in these areas, will also have an impact on the degree of preparedness with which the patient faces the challenges presented by the termination phase.

INDICATIONS FOR TERMINATION

The indications for termination of DPHP are determined by the treatment goals established at the beginning of treatment. When these goals have been attained, or approximated sufficiently to meet the patient's satisfaction, and when these gains are stable, it is time to consider termination. Symptomatic improvement as a result of treatment should correspond with personality change (i.e., decreased personality rigidity) in areas of functioning linked to the patient's presenting complaints. Using decreased personality rigidity along with the treatment goals as criteria for termination will distinguish true therapeutic gains from "transference cure," in which there is symptomatic improvement in the absence of personality change. In the case of transference cure, the patient's improvement is contingent upon ongoing contact with the therapist, whereas gains reflecting personality change are relatively stable and will be sustained, or may even continue to develop, after termination.

Many, if not most, patients become transiently symptomatic at some point in the termination phase and may appear to lose many of the gains that have been made in treatment. This apparent regression should be managed as a relatively routine aspect of the working through of the termination phase and not necessarily as an indication to reconsider ending the treatment.

TIMING OF TERMINATION

The topic of termination may be introduced by either the patient or the therapist. Some patients raise this topic throughout the course of treatment. When they do so prematurely, their comments typically reflect reactions to object relations activated in the transference. The patient's premature suggestion to end the treatment should be explored and analyzed, just as any other clinical material would be.

In contrast, in the latter portions of the middle phase, when treatment goals have been met to a significant degree, it becomes appropriate to discuss termination in realistic terms. It is important that the DPHP therapist keep in mind that, regardless of whether it is the patient or the therapist who raises the topic, and even if the patient is comfortable that it is time to end the treatment, discussion of termination as a real possibility will stir up reactions in the patient. Before moving ahead and setting a date for ending, patient and therapist will do well to explore what it means to the patient to end the treatment, with particular attention to the transference fantasies linked to this discussion.

We recommend setting a termination date at least 3 months, and no more than 6 months, in advance of the actual ending, with longer treatments benefiting from a longer termination phase. Less than 3 months is often not enough time to optimally consolidate gains and work through the issues stimulated by ending treatment. On the other hand, if a date is set too far in advance, the prospect of termination becomes so distant that the patient cannot realistically focus on ending.

ANALYSIS OF SEPARATIONS DURING TREATMENT

Analysis of the patient's responses to separations from the therapist during weekends, vacations, and illnesses during the course of treatment will predict the patient's reactions to termination. Patients' responses to separation from the therapist can be described along a spectrum of degrees of integration—from paranoid, to depressive, through normal. Normal reactions to separation from the therapist include sadness, a sense of loss, and mourning. Depending on the circumstances, a normal reaction to separation may also include a sense of freedom, of well-being, and a looking ahead to the future.

Depressive reactions to separation are dominated by intense sadness and idealization of the therapist, often in conjunction with feelings of guilt, unworthiness, and a tendency to cling to the relationship. Fantasies of being responsible for having driven the therapist away or worn him out are common.

In contrast, paranoid responses to separation from the therapist are marked by severe separation anxiety, so that, instead of sadness, the patient experiences intense anxiety and fear of abandonment. There is a tendency to see the therapist as a "bad" object who is abandoning, attacking, or frustrating the patient.

During the course of treatment, the therapist explores the patient's reactions to interruptions in the treatment. Repetitive analysis of these reactions will move the patient from a more paranoid or depressive reaction and toward a normal one and will prepare him for termination. When patients present with a mix of paranoid and depressive reactions to separation, paranoid reactions should be analyzed before depressive ones; as discussed earlier, analysis of paranoid object relations will facilitate more complete and successful working through of depressive conflicts. In DPHP, paranoid elements in the patient's reactions to separations can sometimes provide an opportunity to explore and work through more "primitive" object relations that may otherwise be too deeply repressed to access in treatment.

CLINICAL ILLUSTRATIONS OF ANXIETIES STIMULATED BY SEPARATION FROM THE THERAPIST

As an example of the unearthing of repressed paranoid object relations in a patient with higher level personality pathology in response to separation from the therapist, we describe a vignette from the treatment of a mildly depressed young woman who presented with severe sexual inhibitions and problems with self-esteem. In treatment, depressive conflicts around competitive sexual and aggressive themes were enacted and analyzed. The therapist made interpretations in relation to the patient's guilt about imagined oedipal triumphs and her defensive need to see herself in a devalued fashion. The therapist saw little overt evidence of paranoid object relations in the opening phase of the treatment.

Some 10 months into treatment, the therapist took a planned 4-week vacation. About halfway through this break period the patient became acutely paranoid in relation to her husband. She experienced him as selfish and callous, someone who exploited her and had no concern for her welfare. She found herself enraged. Yet at the same time she was aware that her feelings were not reasonable and that they were different from anything she had experienced during 5 years of a relatively happy marriage.

Upon the therapist's return, it became possible to analyze the object relation of a callous and selfish maternal figure in relation to a hateful child, which had been activated by the therapist's leaving. This paranoid object relation, which was seen to underlie the patient's conflicts around competition, had been entirely unconscious until activated by separation from the therapist. Working through the paranoid concerns that had been activated by the therapist's leaving facilitated subsequent successful working through of oedipal conflicts.

As an example of a normal reaction to separation, we describe another patient, one approaching the end of a successful treatment. He began talking about ending the treatment several months before his therapist's summer vacation. A date for ending had not yet been set, but the patient continued to feel that he wanted to wrap things up. On the eve of his therapist's vacation, the patient noted that although he anticipated missing the therapist and the treatment as he had done during interruptions of the treatment in the past, he felt less fearful and less needy about it. In some ways he was looking forward to the opportunity to see what it felt like not to have the therapist to lean on, and because he usually saw his therapist in the early morning, he also was pleasurably anticipating more leisurely mornings in bed with his girlfriend.

In contrast, during the therapist's vacation the previous summer, this same patient had been aware of feeling needy before the therapist left, and he had had the thought that the therapist might be looking forward to a welcome break from the patient's "whining." Over that break, the patient had felt depressed and self-critical and was convinced that he was doing a bad job at his work. The connection between these affects and the therapist's absence had not been evident to the patient until the therapist pointed it out upon his return.

SEPARATION AT THE END OF TREATMENT

By the time the patient with higher level personality pathology approaches termination, therapist and patient will have had many opportunities to analyze the patient's responses to separations from the therapist. Typically, in DPHP, we see a mix of normal and depressive reactions to termination. Depressive reactions to termination should be systematically analyzed and worked through over the course of months before ending treatment. We do not recommend terminating treatment if the patient's experience of separations remains predominantly paranoid. Although transient paranoid reactions to termination are not uncommon, persistent and predominant paranoid reactions to separations are indications for further working through of paranoid anxieties in ongoing treatment.

Thus far, we have focused on patients' typical reactions to separation from the therapist at termination from the perspective of loss. However, typical reactions to termination of DPHP involve not only the experience of loss but also reactions to success. It is common, if not universal, for patients ending successful treatments to entertain at least fleeting concerns that they are somehow hurting the therapist by leaving. Patients may imagine that the therapist will be left feeling lonely, left behind, or old in the patient's absence or that the therapist is dependent on income from the patient and will be financially burdened by the patient's successfully moving on. Analyzing these fantasies during the termination phase provides a final opportunity to work through depressive conflicts in the transference and will help to consolidate gains made in treatment.

AMBIVALENCE IN THE TERMINATION PHASE

In addition to noting and consolidating gains, patients in the termination phase of DPHP must also consider what has not been accomplished in the treatment. They must acknowledge and mourn not only loss of the therapist but also loss of an ideal version of what it was hoped would be accomplished in treatment. Even when treatment goals are successfully met, the

patient in the termination phase is confronted with the reality that his personality and his behavior remain less than perfect. The capacity to work
through both the disappointments and the gains of a successful DPHP
treatment implies that the patient has attained a comfortably integrated
sense of himself.

Working through disappointments also involves facing disappointment
in the therapist and in the treatment. The capacity to entertain a generally
positive view of the therapist while maintaining awareness of his limitations
implies an ambivalent attitude on the part of the patient toward the therapist. In a successful termination, feelings of disappointment and resentment
can be contained within an overall positive view of the therapeutic relationship, characterized by a sense of genuine appreciation for the therapist's
skill and gratitude for the help the therapist has provided.

MAINTAINING THE TREATMENT FRAME THROUGH TERMINATION

We recommend maintaining a twice-weekly frame through the end of
treatment. Wishes on the part of the patient or the therapist to taper sessions or to "wean" the patient from treatment reflect the desire to mitigate
anxieties stimulated by ending treatment and separating from the therapist.
In DPHP, this is exactly what we do not want to do; rather, we want to allow
these anxieties to emerge so that they can be explored and worked through.
This process makes it easier for the patient to function well without the
therapist in the post-termination phase, and it also provides an important
opportunity to consolidate treatment gains.

We also recommend maintaining the therapeutic relationship, without
abandoning technical neutrality or changing the way therapist and patient
interact, as the treatment comes to an end. Having said this, we add that it
is inevitable that the relationship between patient and therapist will take on
a more realistic quality as treatment comes to an end and transferences are
worked through. However, beyond this natural evolution in the therapeutic
relationship, we do not recommend that the therapist change his role or assume a more socially friendly or openly supportive stance in relation to the
patient during the final weeks of treatment. In final sessions, it is appropriate
for the therapist to mark the gains that have been made and to communicate
whatever positive feelings he has about having worked with the patient.

THERAPIST REACTIONS TO PATIENT TERMINATION

It is natural for a therapist to experience a mourning reaction at the ending
of a DPHP treatment—particularly one that has been especially long or

rewarding. In addition, depressive concerns on the part of therapists are not uncommon at termination. As patients voice and work through their disappointment in the treatment, it is not uncommon for therapists to feel guilty. Feelings of regret or self-criticism—such as that the therapist could have done a better job or that perhaps someone else might have—are particularly common among inexperienced therapists. Like the patient, the therapist must come to terms with what was not accomplished in the treatment.

PREMATURE TERMINATION

Some patients want to end treatment before the treatment goals have been attained. In this situation, the therapist should explore the patient's motivations for leaving and link them to anxieties currently being activated in the treatment, paying special attention to the transference. If the patient persists in wanting to leave, the therapist should share a realistic assessment of what has been accomplished, what has not been accomplished, and what could be expected from further work.

If the patient persists in wanting to end the treatment prematurely, the therapist should avoid engaging in a power struggle. It is appropriate for the therapist to frankly share his reservations about ending at this time and then to establish a mutually agreed-upon date to stop meeting, ideally at least a month in advance. The therapist can explain to the patient that it is helpful to establish this time period for wrapping things up and consolidating gains. The therapist should also explain that "the door is open" should the patient feel that he would like to pursue treatment at some point in the future.

POST-TERMINATION CONTACT

If the patient does not raise the question of future contact between therapist and patient after ending treatment, it is appropriate for the therapist to do so. It is not uncommon for patients to believe that they are not "supposed" or "allowed" to contact the therapist in the future or that doing so would indicate a failure of the treatment. The therapist should communicate that he is available to the patient and would be happy to hear from him in the future, should the need arise.

Some patients will ask about getting together with the therapist socially, for example, meeting him for lunch, after the treatment has ended. We strongly recommend that the DPHP therapist avoid engaging in a social relationship with patients after termination.

THERAPEUTIC IMPASSE

Some treatments do not proceed to termination. Instead, they seem to bog down at some point in the middle phase. Sometimes, therapist and patient come to feel like they are locked into some fundamental disagreement or miscommunication that cannot be successfully analyzed and worked through. At other times, what initially appears to be working through comes to feel like going in circles; the same material comes up repeatedly and may be explored, but this process does not lead anywhere new and the treatment does not progress. It is not unusual for situations of this kind to arise during the course of treatment and to last for several sessions or even for several weeks. However, if the situation persists over a period of months, we begin to think in terms of a "therapeutic impasse."

COMMON CAUSES OF THERAPEUTIC IMPASSE

It is necessary for the therapist to diagnose the root cause of an extended therapeutic impasse before deciding how to proceed. Sometimes, an impasse reflects a chronic transference-countertransference enactment that has not been identified by the therapist or sufficiently worked through (Schlesinger 2005). As a result, the same object relations are enacted over and over again as a way to avoid activation of underlying conflicts—to the detriment of the progress of the treatment. Other common causes of therapeutic impasses in DPHP are undiagnosed, incorrectly diagnosed, or inadequately treated Axis I disorders and incorrect diagnosis of the patient's level of personality organization. Undiagnosed secondary gains can also lead to stasis, although this is less commonly encountered in the treatment of patients with higher level personality pathology than in that of patients with more severe personality pathology.

When the psychotherapeutic process is "stuck," it often emerges that chronic countertransferences are interfering with the therapist's ability to diagnose what is actually going on in the treatment. Alternatively, the therapist may accurately understand what is happening but feels in some way constrained in the countertransference, so that he is unable to effectively make use of his understanding to move the treatment along. As a result, if a treatment is stuck over a period of many months and the therapist is unable to clarify the cause of the problem or unable to help the patient work it through, consultation with a colleague is always indicated and is generally very helpful.

SUGGESTED READINGS

Fairbairn R: The repression and the return of bad objects (with special reference to the "War Neuroses") (1943), in Psychoanalytic Studies of Personality. London, Routledge, 1952, pp 59–81

Freud S: Recommendations to physicians practicing psychoanalysis (1912), in The Standard Edition of the Complete Psychological Works of Sigmund Freud, Vol 12. Edited and translated by Strachey J. London, Hogarth Press, 1958, pp 109–120

Gray P: On helping analysands observe intrapsychic activity, in The Ego and Analysis of Defense, 2nd Edition. New York, Jason Aronson, 2005, pp 63–86

Klein M: On the criteria for terminating a psycho-analysis. Int J Psychoanal 31:78–80, 1950

Rosenfeld H: Negative therapeutic reaction. Reported in the transactions of the Topeka Analytic Society. Bull Menninger Clin 34:180–192, 1970

Sandler J, Dare C, Holder H: The negative therapeutic reaction, in The Patient and the Analyst, 2nd Edition. Madison, CT, International Universities Press, 1992, pp 121–132

Schafer R: The termination of brief psychoanalytic psychotherapy. International Journal of Psychoanalytic Psychotherapy 2:135–148, 1973

Schlesinger HJ: Endings and Beginnings: On Terminating Psychotherapy and Psychoanalysis. Hillsdale, NJ, Analytic Press, 2005

COMBINING DPHP WITH MEDICATION MANAGEMENT AND OTHER FORMS OF TREATMENT

Patients with higher level personality pathology who are seen in consultation may present with a variety of symptoms or relational problems. In particular, symptoms of depression and anxiety, marital problems, sexual symptoms, and various forms of substance misuse are common. Because dynamic psychotherapy for higher level personality pathology (DPHP) is not a treatment for specific symptoms or DSM-IV-TR Axis I disorders (American Psychiatric Association 2000), these patients require careful diagnostic assessment to determine whether there are indications for psychopharmacological intervention or a symptom-oriented or problem-oriented psychotherapy, either instead of or in combination with DPHP. Depending on the nature of the patient's difficulties, DPHP can at times be advantageously combined with medication management, couples therapy, sexual therapy, group therapy, behavior therapy, cognitive-behavioral therapy (CBT), and 12-step programs.

In this chapter we focus on the management of patients who present with *both* clinically significant higher level personality pathology *and* an Axis I disorder or relational problems that may warrant specific attention. We focus primarily on strategies for combining DPHP with psychopharmacological management of depression. In addition we cover the management of patients with anxiety disorders, and we comment briefly on combining DPHP with other forms of psychotherapy for marital, sexual, and interpersonal problems.

COMBINING DPHP WITH TREATMENTS FOR DEPRESSION

A large proportion of patients with higher level personality pathology seen in consultation complain of "depression." The differential diagnosis for patients presenting with complaints of depressed mood include major depression, dysthymia, depression not otherwise specified, bipolar disorders, adjustment reactions with depressed mood, pathological mourning reactions, depression secondary to medical illness, chronic dysphoria as part of a DSM-IV-TR personality disorder, and depressive affect associated with higher level personality pathology.

If, during initial consultation, a patient endorses depressive symptoms, the therapist-consultant should do a careful evaluation for depressive illness. Not uncommonly, patients will present with a complex combination of affective illness, comorbid personality rigidity, and significant psychosocial stressors, all of which appear to be contributing to the patient's current depressed mood. However, regardless of the therapist's impression with regard to the etiology of the patient's depressive symptoms, the diagnosis of affective illness is made on the basis of the descriptive features of the patient's illness.

Depression tends to recur, and adequate and timely treatment reduces the risk of recurrence (Dubovsky et al. 2003). As a result, when a patient receives diagnoses of depressive illness *and* higher level personality pathology, management of depression is the highest immediate clinical priority. When the diagnostic impression is of DSM-IV-TR major depression or dysthymia in conjunction with clinically significant personality rigidity, the therapist should share this impression with the patient, review the treatment options, and, together with the patient, formulate a treatment plan.

A variety of treatments have demonstrated efficacy for major depression and dysthymia. In addition to antidepressant medications, a number of symptom-oriented psychotherapies have been developed for and shown to be effective in the treatment of depression. CBT is the psychotherapy for depression that has been most widely studied, but interpersonal therapy

(IPT) and, to a lesser extent, short-term dynamic psychotherapy (STDP) have also been shown to be effective (Beutler et al. 2000; Lambert and Ogles 2004; Leichsenring 2001).

In contrast to antidepressant medication and symptom-oriented psychotherapies, DPHP has not been systematically studied as a treatment for affective illness, and there are few empirical data to support its effectiveness. On this basis, we do not recommend DPHP as a treatment for depression until standard treatment options have been exhausted. At the same time, treatments for depression are not designed to treat personality rigidity. As a result, for the patient with depressive illness in the context of clinically significant higher level personality rigidity, we generally recommend combining antidepressant medication with DPHP.

TREATING DEPRESSIVE DISORDERS: SEQUENTIAL TREATMENT

When treating the patient who presents with depressive illness in the setting of clinically significant higher level personality pathology, we recommend sequential treatment. Specifically, we recommend initiating treatment of depression before addressing underlying personality pathology. We make this recommendation, in part, because what appears to be personality rigidity may improve as affective symptoms resolve (Dubovsky et al. 2003). In other cases, the patient is satisfied once affective illness is treated, because personality rigidity either is relatively mild or is not troubling to the patient. Alternatively, in cases where personality rigidity *is* clinically significant, as depressive symptoms resolve, patient and therapist can see more clearly the ways in which personality rigidity and maladaptive behavior patterns continue to cause distress and interfere with the patient's functioning and life satisfaction. In this situation, as affective symptoms improve, it becomes appropriate to identify specific treatment goals and begin a course of DPHP.

The goal of medication management is to either obtain full remission of symptoms or achieve the best possible medication response. Because fewer than 50% of depressed patients achieve remission with the first selective serotonin reuptake inhibitor (SSRI) prescribed (Thase et al. 2001), many patients will require ongoing medication management that involves either switching medication or augmenting the original treatment prescribed. Furthermore, when medication has been prescribed and there has been a partial response, one cannot assume that residual symptoms of depression reflect personality rigidity until a systematic psychopharmacological strategy has been exhausted. As a result, sequential treatment will not infrequently entail starting a program of medication trials, obtaining partial remission of symptoms, and beginning DPHP while continuing to optimize medication management of depressive symptoms.

The alternative to sequential treatment of depressive illness and higher level personality pathology is to establish treatment goals and begin DPHP while simultaneously beginning pharmacological treatment for depression. The problem with this approach is that treatment goals may change or even disappear as depression remits. Furthermore, depressed patients are often unable to make full use of DPHP and will do better with a more structured psychotherapeutic approach geared toward symptom management until affective symptoms begin to remit.

When sequential treatment is initiated, medication can be prescribed by the DPHP therapist (if he is a psychiatrist) while seeing the patient in weekly or biweekly sessions. In these sessions, therapist and patient can get to know one another and can begin to establish a working alliance while focusing on coping with depression, symptom management, and monitoring medication side effects and treatment response. In the case of uncomplicated depression that responds to an SSRI, as symptoms of depression remit, goals for DPHP can be established and a course of therapy initiated.

If the patient does not want to take medication and symptoms are not severe, CBT, IPT, and STDP are alternatives to medication management. In this setting, after completing a course of therapy for depression, the clinician and patient can reassess the need and the patient's motivation for DPHP.

When starting to work with a patient for whom specific treatment for depression and DPHP are both apparently indicated, it is important that the therapist be explicit with the patient about the different goals for the two treatment approaches, the different ways that the treatments work, and the differences between the symptom-oriented therapy that typically accompanies the initial phases of medication management on the one hand and DPHP on the other—including the role and stance of the therapist and the time frame for the treatment. In cases in which depression is remitting on medication and a course of DPHP is initiated, the shift to DPHP should be made explicit. Changes will involve moving to twice-weekly sessions, revising treatment goals, and introducing the respective roles of therapist and patient in the psychotherapeutic relationship. As part of obtaining informed consent for treatment, the therapist should explain that DPHP does not have demonstrated efficacy for treatment of affective illness, whereas antidepressant medication, CBT, IPT, and STDP do meet this criterion.

CLINICAL ILLUSTRATION OF SEQUENTIAL TREATMENT

A 39-year-old married college professor requested "insight-oriented psychotherapy" 2 months after having been passed over for academic promotion. In the initial consultation, the patient described himself as "swamped" by self-recriminations and "unable to cope" with his feelings of failure and disappointment. In addition, he was isolating himself socially and complained of poor appetite and insomnia. The patient had had a similar episode while in college that was successfully treated with antidepressant medication.

After careful evaluation, the therapist made the diagnosis of major depressive disorder, recurrent. She explained to the patient that she thought he was depressed, that this was a recurrence of what had happened in college, and that his symptoms would likely respond to medication. She also explained that DPHP is not a treatment designed to treat depression but if he preferred therapy over medication, she could refer him to a colleague for CBT. The therapist also shared her impression that the patient might have other areas of difficulty—areas related to his personality that were not attributable to depression—that might well benefit from DPHP, but that it was difficult to make this assessment with certainty while he was depressed. She suggested that he be treated for depression and then reevaluated for possible indications for DPHP.

The patient agreed to a trial of medication while meeting weekly with the therapist. In weekly sessions, the therapist evaluated the patient for medication response and side effects. She also encouraged him to use the time to help her get to know him better and to develop a better understanding of the events that had occurred around the time of the onset of his depression. Initially, the patient focused on his feelings of depression and agitation and on his difficulty in coping with self-recriminations. The therapist listened sympathetically, suggested to the patient that his self-critical thoughts were being exacerbated by the depression, and reminded him that he should be feeling the benefit of the medication shortly. As the patient began to feel less agitated and depressed, he began to talk more about areas of his life that were sources of frustration. In these sessions, the therapist noted that the patient, now less depressed, was able to talk about his recent academic difficulties in a more reflective and less aggressively self-critical fashion than in the initial consultation.

After having been on medication for 6 weeks, the patient came into a session saying that he had realized he was feeling much better, almost his "usual self." He remained disappointed about having been passed over for promotion but was hopeful that he might be promoted the following year. At the same time, he was putting out feelers for openings at other colleges in the area. The patient also reflected on his inability to deal with the perceived failure at the time that he first came to the therapist. He felt that this was somewhat out of character; although a perfectionist, he had weathered previous disappointments with much greater equanimity. He attributed his difficulty, to some degree, to his depression.

The therapist told the patient that she shared his impression that his depression seemed to be remitting. She went on to say that this raised the question of whether there were more chronic aspects of his personality or functioning that were troubling to him or if things felt pretty much okay. The patient responded that although he was feeling better and more self-confident, their exploration of the events leading up to his failed promotion had left him concerned about ways in which he might have contributed to his professional setbacks, both recently and in the past.

For the first time, the patient acknowledged to the therapist his awareness that he had not handled departmental politics effectively in recent months, even though he had known this could affect his possibilities for promotion. On hearing this, the therapist remembered the patient describing how, despite an overall record of success in many areas of his life, he had had a propensity since adolescence to always come in second, never winning first place. The therapist suggested to the patient that there might be a link between this piece of history and his behavior in his professional life, and she suggested that perhaps he had complicated feelings about competing and winning. The patient acknowledged having wondered about that himself, and he shared a concern that his apparent difficulty with winning had led to subtle forms of self-sabotage that might have limited his professional advancement over the years.

The therapist suggested to the patient that his difficulty with competition was something he could work on in DPHP if he were motivated to do so. The therapist explained her understanding of how DPHP could be helpful to him. After the therapist answered the patient's questions about the treatment, he expressed interest in proceeding. Together, patient and therapist established treatment goals and agreed to begin meeting twice weekly.

The therapist explained to the patient that they would, to some degree, be making a change in the role that each had played in the sessions up to that point. She encouraged him to allow his mind to wander freely and to discuss whatever came to mind in a less structured way than he had been doing when his attention had been largely focused on his depression. She also explained that he might find her to be more reflective and to some degree less active than she had been in the earlier parts of the treatment, as she focused on helping him deepen his understanding of his inner life. The therapist added that even though they would be less focused on his depression per se, both patient and therapist would need to be alert to possible signs of a recurrence of depressive symptoms or the need to make changes in his medication.

BEYOND SEQUENTIAL TREATMENT: MEDICATION MANAGEMENT DURING DPHP

When a patient who is in DPHP is also taking antidepressant medication, it is important that the therapist remain cognizant of the status of the patient's depressive symptoms throughout the course of treatment. Many patients will require ongoing adjustment of medication regimen in order to optimize treatment of depressive illness (Rush et al. 2006). Furthermore, even when depressive symptoms are in full remission, it remains necessary to continue to evaluate the patient for long-term side effects of medications and recurrence of symptoms. The need for the therapist to keep an eye on the course of affective illness applies, regardless of whether the therapist or an outside consultant is prescribing and monitoring medication.

The DPHP therapist who is monitoring the course and treatment of his patient's affective illness faces conflicting demands as he listens to his patient, evaluates what is going on in the treatment, and formulates his interventions. In his role as a DPHP therapist who is treating a patient with higher level personality pathology, the therapist listens for the object relations being enacted in the session and thinks in terms of the unconscious meanings, motivations, and defenses embedded in the patient's relatively unstructured communications. In this context, the therapist's interventions aim at deepening the patient's understanding of his inner life. In contrast, in his role as a healthcare provider treating a patient with depressive illness, the therapist listens for and actively inquires about the phenomenology of the patient's symptoms and side effects and thinks in terms of adequate or partial remission of symptoms, side effects, and recurrence. His interventions aim at the amelioration of symptoms and of any side effects.

Listening to the Patient

The DPHP therapist who treats a patient with affective illness is called upon to embrace two very different ways of listening to and interacting with his patient. For a simple example, consider the therapist in session with a patient who is evidently irritable, first complaining about his wife and his friends and ultimately feeling annoyed with the therapist. The DPHP therapist in role will notice and experience the patient's irritability and attempt to clarify the object relations being enacted in the treatment. However, if the patient has an affective illness, the therapist must leave room in his mind to shift frames of reference and consider whether the patient may be irritable because his affective illness is inadequately treated or because he is having side effects to his medication. The first, psychodynamic frame of reference calls upon the therapist to listen to the patient's associations, explore what he is thinking and feeling, and make an interpretation when appropriate. The second frame of reference, based in phenomenology and a medical model, calls upon the therapist to actively evaluate the patient's symptoms and recommend a change in medication or request a consultation with a pharmacologist when appropriate.

To effectively treat a patient with depressive illness in DPHP, the therapist must be able to hold in mind two very different models of treatment. This calls on the therapist to focus in his own mind on both psychodynamics *and* phenomenology and to alternate between two ways of listening to and thinking about his patient's thoughts, feelings, and behaviors. The need to hold both models in mind applies regardless of whether the therapist is an M.D. and regardless of who is providing medication management.

Early in treatment, when management of depression is often more active, the situation may call upon the therapist to oscillate between the two frames of reference—listening within a psychodynamic framework and circling back to consider phenomenology—and then decide at which level to intervene. Later in treatment, when the management of affective illness is no longer acute, the therapist has greater freedom to focus more consistently on the psychodynamic model of pathology and treatment. However, throughout the course of treatment the DPHP therapist treating the patient with depressive illness must be open to hearing and thinking about the things his patient is saying, doing, and experiencing not only in terms of the patient's psychodynamics and underlying personality organization but also as manifestations of the patient's affective illness.

Intervening

The patient with affective illness will not spontaneously tell the therapist everything he needs to know about symptoms and side effects. As a result, the therapist must make active and systematic inquiry about the course of affective illness, not only in the initial consultation or opening phase but also at various times throughout the course of treatment. The need to provide ongoing evaluation and management of affective illness during DPHP will call upon the therapist to at times interact with his patient in a way that is more structured and more directive than is typical for the DPHP therapist in role, by setting the agenda and systematically asking the patient to provide specific information. When a therapist anticipates the need to initiate interactions with a DPHP patient regarding symptoms and medication management, it is generally best to do so at the beginning of a session whenever possible. However, a patient may bring the management of affective illness to center stage at any point in a session, either directly, by describing symptoms or side effects, or indirectly, by revealing aspects of his experience or behavior that in the therapist's mind warrant further evaluation.

In the same way that the DPHP therapist treating patients with affective illness must shift between two different ways of listening to his patient, he must also shift back and forth between two different ways of interacting with him in acquiring data and intervening. However, in contrast to when the therapist shifts frames of references as he listens to the patient, when the therapist shifts between two ways of intervening, it will be immediately noticeable to the patient. In addition, although it may be tempting to consider interactions around affective illness to be "medical" and therefore somehow "not part of the therapy," this is a distinction that does not exist in the unconscious mind of the patient—nor in that of the therapist, for that matter.

Interactions regarding management of affective illness will have an impact on the transference and typically on the countertransference as well. As a result, as he interacts with his patient around medication management, the DPHP therapist must remain mindful that he is participating in enactments that will have specific meanings to the patient, based on the patient's dynamics and what has been going on in treatment. Enactments related to management of affective illness should be handled as one would any other form of enactment; the therapist should be ready to explore the patient's experience of the object relations embedded in their exchanges. When a pharmacologist is involved, exploration of the patient's reactions to the pharmacologist will often shed light on the object relations being enacted in the treatment as well, as those that are being defended against.

CLINICAL ILLUSTRATION OF ISSUES RAISED BY MEDICATION MANAGEMENT DURING DPHP

A 55-year-old professional woman had been in DPHP for 6 months with a male therapist who had recently graduated from training. On initial presentation, the patient had been depressed and was started on an SSRI, with which she achieved full remission of her symptoms.

The patient came into a session on Monday morning, was silent for a time, and then began to complain of feeling "fat and unattractive." The therapist wondered if the patient's view of herself as unattractive was a retreat from the erotic atmosphere that he had sensed toward the end of the previous session. Simultaneously, the therapist looked at the patient and noticed for the first time that she had, indeed, gained a fair amount of weight.

The therapist inquired about the weight gain. The patient told him that she had gained 10 pounds over a period of a couple of months. She went on to say that she had never had a weight problem before, but this time she just could not take off the weight. The therapist raised the possibility that the patient's weight gain might be related to the medication she was taking. She responded that she had done a fair amount of research online over the previous month, and she thought it very likely that the medication was responsible for her weight problem. The therapist discussed treatment options with the patient, and they decided to switch to a different antidepressant that was less likely to cause weight gain. They also agreed that the patient would weigh herself weekly and share this information with the therapist.

The therapist realized that he felt uneasy and somehow guilty. He found himself thinking that he should have more actively inquired about potential long-term side effects, and he was troubled by his failure to have noticed the patient's weight gain earlier. He was also struck by the fact that the patient had been researching the side effects of antidepressants for quite some time without mentioning this to the therapist. The therapist asked her about it. The patient responded that she had felt guilty bringing it up with the therapist. The medication had really helped her, and she did not want to make him feel bad; as they explored the patient's concerns, it became apparent that she feared if she were to talk about side effects, the therapist would feel criticized. They identified an object relation of an easily angered and narcissistically vulnerable parent who needs to be in control interacting with a child who tries to please. This object relation helped the patient to remain unaware of her own critical feelings toward the therapist. To "complain" was both guilt-provoking and risky because it threatened to bring her into contact with these unacceptable, aggressive feelings.

The therapist then reflected on why the patient had raised the topic of her weight in this particular session. He wondered if the object relation they had explored, reflecting the patient's anxiety about causing the therapist to feel criticized by her, was defending against erotic feelings and anxiety about causing him to feel sexually excited by her. Perhaps the patient's reluctance to raise the issue of her weight reflected anxiety about calling the therapist's attention to her body. The therapist then thought about his own guilty feelings earlier in the session. It occurred to him that his failure to notice the patient's weight gain might reflect his own anxiety about focusing on the body of a woman so close in age to that of his mother. Perhaps he was uncomfortable with the emerging erotic transference-countertransference to a degree that he had not been fully aware of.

DEPRESSION EMERGING DURING DPHP

Some patients who begin DPHP have a history of depressive illness but are not currently depressed when starting treatment. Some will be on maintenance or prophylactic medication. Because affective illness tends to recur (Dubovsky et al. 2003), it is not uncommon for patients in this group, particularly those who are not on medication, to become depressed during the course of treatment. As a result, when treating patients with a history of affective illness, the therapist must remain mindful of the possibility of recurrence throughout the course of therapy. In addition, during the consultation phase and before beginning DPHP with a patient with a history of affective illness, it is wise to discuss the possibility of recurrence with the patient.

If, during the course of DPHP, the therapist or the patient becomes concerned that the patient may be becoming depressed, this calls for careful and systematic evaluation of symptoms. If the therapist's diagnosis is recurrence of depressive illness, the therapist should first clearly explain to the patient what has led him to conclude that the patient may be becoming depressed and then discuss treatment options with the patient. When antidepressant medication is initiated or adjusted during the course of DPHP, it is important to address what the addition of medication and medication management to the treatment means to the patient.

CLINICAL ILLUSTRATION OF DEPRESSION EMERGING DURING DPHP

A professional woman presented shortly before her thirtieth birthday complaining of anxiety related to concerns that she would never be married. She told the therapist-consultant that she was interested in better understanding why she had been unable to become engaged despite having sustained several long-term relationships.

At initial presentation, she seemed anxious and preoccupied. She described difficulty sleeping and a tendency to sit in bed at night with anxious thoughts about becoming "a spinster in a rocking chair, surrounded by cats." She denied other symptoms of depression, and she explained that she did not view herself as depressed. Although the patient was animated and demonstrated a full range of emotion during the consultation, the therapist noted that she cried several times during the course of her first visit. The patient's mother had had depression, but the patient herself had never been treated for depression. Her father had been killed in a car accident when the patient was 18 months old.

The therapist explained to the patient that it seemed she had at least one problem, and possibly two. First, as the patient herself had noted, she seemed to have problems with intimate relationships, particularly with making a long-term commitment to a man. The therapist suggested that even though she had had seemingly rational reasons for breaking it off with each boyfriend, it was possible that there were also less rational motivations outside of her awareness that might be guiding her behavior and interfering with her making a commitment to a partner. The therapist explained that DPHP was a treatment that could help her gain a clearer understanding of what was motivating her behavior, with the aim of enabling her to make good choices for herself in the future.

The therapist went on to say that she thought the patient might have another problem as well. The patient did not view herself as depressed, but from the therapist's perspective, the patient's sense of panic, her anxious ruminations, and her easy tearfulness suggested the patient was becoming depressed. In light of the family history, this was a real possibility. The therapist went on to explain that if indeed the patient were to become depressed, it would likely require specific treatment; DPHP would not necessarily be sufficient.

The patient was quite adamant that she did not feel depressed. She told the therapist that just the decision to seek treatment had left her feeling better, and she was sure that if she got into a good relationship and made a commitment, she would feel fine. She had seen her mother's recurrent depressions and knew that she did not feel the way her mother did. The therapist acknowledged her own uncertainty as to whether the patient's anxiety and tearfulness represented a transient reaction to her life situation and upcoming birthday—a situation that would resolve on its own—or whether they were seeing prodromal symptoms of an emerging depressive episode that would require treatment. They discussed the options and agreed to begin DPHP while continuing to keep an eye on the patient's mood. The patient remained adamant that she was not depressed and would feel fine if she had a boyfriend.

Over the next 6 weeks, the therapist noted that during the patient's twice-weekly sessions, she was not able to speak freely or really to talk about anything in session other than her panic about never getting married, and this situation did not change over time. The patient was visibly anxious and, over the weeks, became increasingly tearful. The therapist noticed that the patient appeared to be losing weight, and she began to allude to not wanting to socialize and to feeling marginalized at work. At this point, the therapist again raised the issue of depression and shared with the patient her impression both that the patient seemed to be depressed and also that she seemed frightened to acknowledge this as a possibility.

In response, the patient began to talk about her fear of becoming disabled by mental illness, as her mother had been. The therapist pointed out that being depressed did not mean that the patient had to be disabled; her mother had always refused treatment, and it was very likely that, if the patient were to allow herself to be treated, her symptoms would remit. Given the patient's complex feelings about pursuing treatment for depression, the therapist recommended a consultation with a colleague of hers, an expert pharmacologist highly attuned to psychodynamic issues who could provide a diagnostic evaluation and offer a second opinion. The patient agreed, and the consultant made the diagnosis of major depressive disorder associated with prominent anxiety; she also tactfully and empathically explored the patient's anxiety about medication. In the end, the patient agreed to a trial of an SSRI, which the therapist prescribed.

The patient continued to see the therapist twice weekly. The content of her sessions moved from her panic about marriage to her fear of having her mother's illness and of being incapacitated as her mother had been. Within 2 months her anxiety abated, and she was less tearful. She began to assume a more realistic attitude toward her future; she recognized both that at the age of 30, she still had time to marry and start a family and that her affective illness did not need to follow the same destructive course that had characterized her mother's illness.

As the patient became less anxious and depressed, and at the same time more accepting of having an affective illness, she also became more self-reflective. Therapist and patient agreed that the patient, now on medication, could benefit from DPHP. They reframed the goal of the treatment in terms of understanding the motivations underlying her failure to get married, in particular as these motivations related to her complex feelings toward her chronically depressed mother.

"SPLIT" TREATMENT

A psychiatrist treating a patient with higher level personality pathology and current affective illness in DPHP faces the question of whether to "split" the treatment with another therapist or a pharmacologist or to wear both hats himself, functioning as pharmacologist and therapist for the patient. This is a complex decision that is best made on a case-by-case basis. Although there are always exceptions to generalizations, in our experience with patients with higher level personality pathology simultaneously treated with medication management and DPHP, when medication response is robust and side effects are few, there is no need to split the treatment in this way. In contrast, as medication management becomes more complex and time consuming, requiring various medication trials to optimize response, it may become desirable to involve a pharmacologist. In practice, most psychiatrists function as both pharmacologists and therapists with their therapy patients, whereas non-M.D. therapists have no choice but to offer split treatment.

There are advantages and disadvantages both to split treatments and to treatments provided by a single clinician. The advantages of a single clinician functioning as therapist and pharmacologist are in part practical—the patient is spared the expense of seeing two professionals, and the therapist is spared the time needed to maintain ongoing telephone contact with the other caregiver. From a clinical perspective, combined treatment provided by a single clinician will usually make it easier to analyze the transferential implications of medication management. Patients will have transferences to a pharmacologist that may be split off from other transferences to the therapist. When both sets of transferences are activated in relation to a single clinician, it may be easier for the therapist to bring both sets of feelings into the treatment, where they can be worked through.

In addition, from the perspective of optimizing medication management, a therapist-pharmacologist who meets with the patient twice weekly is potentially at an advantage because he may consistently, and in a timely fashion, obtain information relevant to decisions about medication management, including how the patient is doing, the presence of side effects, and the relationship between fluctuations in symptoms and events in the patient's life and in treatment. However, this can be a double-edged sword; the psychiatrist filling the roles of both pharmacologist and therapist will only acquire this information if he systematically asks.

Side by side with the advantages of a single clinician functioning as therapist and pharmacologist are the significant challenges faced by the clinician playing both roles. As we have already discussed, in order to function as both therapist and pharmacologist, a clinician must alternate between two very different ways of listening to and intervening with a patient. From the perspective of the therapy, there is a risk of the therapist's turning to a medical model to the neglect of dynamic themes that are being enacted in the treatment. From the perspective of pharmacology, there is a risk of the therapist's feeling too constrained by his role as therapist to focus consistently and thoroughly on medical management.

Although split treatments have advantages and will, regardless, be standard practice among non-psychiatrists, split treatments present the therapist with the additional challenges inherent in being part of a treatment team. Specifically, when someone other than the therapist is responsible for medication management, it falls to the therapist to keep himself abreast of the course and management of the patient's affective illness, to establish and maintain an open line of communication with the pharmacologist, and to manage transferences that are split between therapist and pharmacologist. These challenges become more difficult to manage when a therapist has mixed feelings about involving a pharmacologist or about the need to move beyond a purely psychodynamic model of treatment. The challenges inherent in any split treatment can be most effectively and satisfactorily managed by frequent and ongoing contact between a therapist who is philosophically and clinically comfortable with psychopharmacology and a pharmacologist who has an appreciation and respect for psychodynamics and, in particular, for the role of transference in the patient's relationship with both therapist and pharmacologist.

When treatments are going to be split, we recommend that the therapist establish an ongoing relationship with a pharmacologist who provides medication management for all patients in the therapist's practice. This enables therapist and pharmacologist to develop, over time, an effective and efficient way of working together, educating one another, and organizing their communications.

COMBINING DPHP WITH TREATMENTS FOR ANXIETY DISORDERS

Like depressive symptoms, symptoms of anxiety are common in patients with higher level personality pathology. The differential diagnosis for symptoms of anxiety in this population include panic disorder, generalized anxiety disorder, social phobia, simple phobia (e.g., fear of flying or claustrophobia), obsessive-compulsive disorder, anxiety disorder not otherwise specified, adjustment reaction with anxiety, anxiety secondary to medical illness or medication, and anxiety associated with higher level personality rigidity. If during initial consultation a patient complains of anxiety, the therapist-consultant should do a careful evaluation for anxiety disorders, medical illnesses, and adjustment reactions, along with assessment of personality rigidity and psychosocial stressors.

Our recommendations for managing patients with higher level personality pathology and comorbid anxiety disorders are essentially the same as those we outlined for managing patients with depressive illness, and we comment here only briefly on issues specific to anxiety disorders. We again emphasize the advantages of sequential treatment, beginning with optimizing treatment of anxiety and then reassessing the patient's need of and motivation for dynamic psychotherapy to treat residual personality rigidity.

When a patient presents with an anxiety disorder in the setting of clinically significant higher level personality pathology, the consultant should explain to the patient that there are a variety of medications and cognitive-behavioral treatments that have demonstrated efficacy for specific anxiety disorders. In contrast, DPHP has not been systematically studied as a treatment for anxiety, and existing studies do not provide empirical support for the efficacy of unstructured dynamic psychotherapies for the treatment of anxiety disorders (Hollander and Simeon 2003). At the same time, treatments for anxiety disorders are not designed to treat personality pathology. Even when symptoms of anxiety are treated to remission, interpersonal, professional, or sexual problems resulting from higher level personality pathology may remain a problem warranting additional treatment.

When treating the patient with personality pathology and a comorbid anxiety disorder, it is important that the DPHP therapist keep in mind that DPHP may, transiently, stir up anxiety at particular points in the treatment. As a result, when a patient whose symptoms of anxiety have been well controlled becomes more symptomatic during DPHP, the clinician will need to distinguish between a recurrence of the patient's anxiety disorder requiring specific treatment on the one hand and transient anxiety stimulated by DPHP on the other. In this setting, we find it is often best not to rush to alter management of the patient's anxiety disorder if symptoms of anxiety are not severe. Instead, before making any changes, the clinician can wait to see if symptoms resolve spontaneously over the course of weeks while continuing to assess the severity of the patient's symptoms and exploring the immediate precipitants of the patient's anxiety.

As with treatment of depression in patients with comorbid higher level personality pathology, when symptoms of anxiety are to be managed predominantly with medication, it is our recommendation that decisions about whether to "split" the treatment be made on a case-by-case basis. In contrast, when the treatment plan entails sequential treatment with CBT or behavior therapy for an anxiety disorder followed by DPHP, we recommend that different therapists provide each of the two treatments. If clinically indicated, maintenance CBT or behavior therapy for an anxiety disorder can be continued while the patient is in DPHP.

COMBINING DPHP WITH SEX THERAPY, COUPLES THERAPY, OR GROUP THERAPY

Many patients with higher level personality pathology present with sexual symptoms or marital problems. For some patients in this group, DPHP combined with sex or couples therapy may be an ideal approach. Similarly, patients with higher level personality pathology who present with social inhibitions or poor interpersonal skills may benefit from assertiveness or social skills training, exposure therapy, or group psychotherapy in conjunction with DPHP.

Combining DPHP with these other, more directive forms of psychotherapy enables patients to directly tackle symptoms and maladaptive relational behaviors in a fashion that is focused and solution-oriented while at
the same time exploring the psychological foundations of symptomatic behaviors with the DPHP therapist. For example, a patient can make use of
feedback given to him in group therapy to facilitate exploration in his individual treatment of the psychological conflicts underlying the maladaptive
interpersonal behaviors he is seeking to change. Similarly, anxieties that are
stimulated by sex therapy or assertiveness training can fruitfully be explored
in DPHP. For some patients a combined approach of this kind may be more
effective and more efficient than either treatment alone or even than the
two treatments in sequence. As is the case when treatments are split between a pharmacologist and DPHP therapist, open and regular communication between the patient's therapists is highly advantageous. Patients with
a history of substance misuse who are stably maintaining sobriety through
participation in a 12-step program may benefit from combining ongoing
12-step treatment with DPHP.

SUGGESTED READINGS

Busch F, Auchincloss E: The psychology of prescribing and taking medication, in Psy-
     chodynamic Concepts in General Psychiatry. Edited by Schwartz H, Bleiberg E,
     Weissman S. Washington, DC, American Psychiatric Press, 1995, pp 401–416

Kahn DA: Medication consultation and split treatment during psychotherapy. J Am
     Acad Psychoanal 19:84–91, 1991

Kessler R: Medication and psychotherapy, in Psychotherapy: The Analytic Ap-
     proach. Edited by Aronson M, Scharfman M. Northvale, NJ, Jason Aronson,
     1992, pp 163–182

Roose S: The use of medication in combination with psychoanalytic psychotherapy
     or psychoanalysis, in Psychiatry. Edited by Michels R. Philadelphia, PA, Lip-
     pincott, 1990, pp 1–8

12

CONCLUDING COMMENTS

Dynamic psychotherapy for higher level personality pathology (DPHP) is an outgrowth of *transference-focused psychotherapy* (TFP), and this handbook is intended to serve as a companion to the TFP manual (Clarkin et al. 2006) developed at the Personality Disorders Institute of the New York Presbyterian Hospital, Westchester Division. Whereas DPHP was developed to treat higher level personality pathology, TFP is a psychodynamic treatment for severe personality disorders. Both treatments are twice-weekly dynamic psychotherapies emerging from contemporary psychodynamic object relations theory. Together, the two manuals provide an integrated approach to the psychodynamic treatment of personality pathology, providing strategies for treating personality pathology across a broad spectrum of severity. We encourage readers to acquaint themselves with both manuals. Those interested in learning more about the Personality Disorders Institute can visit our Web site at http://www.borderlinedisorders.com.

DIAGNOSIS, STRUCTURE, AND TREATMENT OF PERSONALITY PATHOLOGY

Our approach to dynamic psychotherapy is not "one size fits all." Rather, our strategy has been to develop treatments tailored to the specific psychopathology and clinical needs of particular, clearly defined patient populations. Careful evaluation of a patient's psychopathology and his psychological assets precedes and drives differential treatment planning.

The construct of "structural" assessment of personality developed by Kernberg (1984) provides an approach to psychodynamic diagnosis that is designed to guide psychotherapeutic treatment planning. This approach to diagnostic assessment evaluates the nature of psychological structures that organize the individual's experience and behavior. Relying on the constructs of internalized object relations and identity, and focusing on the degree of identity consolidation versus identity pathology, clinicians can classify patients according to severity of personality pathology as reflected in their capacity to establish and maintain realistic, stable, and meaningful experiences of themselves and their significant others.

Our approach to treating personality pathology is organized around modifying psychological structures. We expect that changes in psychological structures, focusing on identity and defensive operations, will be reflected in symptomatic and behavioral change as well as in an overall improved sense of well-being and enjoyment of life. Our approach to treating higher level personality pathology, where identity pathology is absent or relatively mild, seeks to integrate conflictual aspects of self experience into an already relatively well-consolidated sense of self. Our approach to treating more severe personality disorders, where identity pathology is clinically significant, seeks to promote identity consolidation. In both treatments, we focus on the patient's dominant internalized relationship patterns, exploring ways in which these patterns organize the patient's experience of himself and of the world.

RESEARCH

Before one can study the effectiveness of a particular treatment, one must be able to ensure that the treatment being studied is actually being delivered (this is referred to as *treatment adherence*) and that it is being delivered in a reasonably competent fashion. The advent of treatment manuals in the 1960s, which provided a detailed description of a particular treatment along with rating scales for treatment adherence and competence, paved the way for a more sophisticated and empirically sound approach to psychotherapy research than had previously been available (Luborsky and DeRubeis 1984).

Although the majority of psychotherapies that have been manualized to date are short-term treatments, the TFP manual has demonstrated the feasibility of manualizing longer-term and more complex psychodynamically based psychotherapies. The TFP manual has been used by our group to study psychotherapeutic treatment of borderline personality disorder

(BPD). In a randomly controlled clinical trial, 90 patients were assigned to 1 year of TFP; dialectical behavior therapy, a cognitive-behavioral treatment for BPD; or a manualized supportive psychotherapy. Patients in all treatment cells made significant gains across a variety of outcome measures of depression, social adjustment, and global functioning. TFP and dialectical behavior therapy, but not supportive psychotherapy, significantly reduced suicidality (Clarkin JF, Levy KN, Lenzenweger MF, Kernberg OF: "The Personality Disorders Institute/Borderline Personality Disorders Research Foundation Randomized Control Trial of Borderline Personality Disorder: Treatment Outcome," 2005; under review). Reflective functioning, a measure closely tied to the capacity to appreciate and understand the nature of internal thoughts and feelings—both one's own and those of others[1]—significantly improved in the TFP group but not in the dialectical behavior therapy or supportive treatment groups (Levy et al. 2006). The complete data analysis from this study will be published shortly, and long-term follow-up of patients is ongoing. We hypothesize that changes in reflective functioning mirror changes in underlying psychological structures in patients with BPD. In particular, we propose that increases in reflective functioning found in this group of patients treated with TFP correlate with changes in internal object relations and amelioration of identity pathology.

We hope that the description of DPHP that we have presented in this volume will facilitate empirical research into the effectiveness of dynamic psychotherapy for treating Cluster C personality disorders and other types of higher level personality pathology, much as the TFP manual has facilitated empirical research investigating dynamic treatments for BPD.

TRAINING

Although we hope that this handbook will be used to study psychotherapy, we expect that it will be used most often for training clinicians. We have found that our approach, which provides an integrated model of psychopathology linked to a clearly defined theory of psychotherapeutic technique and therapeutic change, is very helpful to students of psychodynamic psychotherapy. However, psychotherapy cannot be learned from reading a book, no matter how good the book might be. Careful reading of a textbook or treatment manual is a first step, but ongoing clinical work under the supervision

---

[1]This capacity is referred to as *mentalization*, and deficits in the capacity for mentalization are thought to play a central role in establishing and maintaining the maladaptive personality traits associated with BPD (Bateman and Fonagy 2004).

of a senior clinician is generally needed if a student is to learn how to practice a psychotherapeutic treatment in a competent fashion. We have found that group supervision may afford additional benefits, not only optimizing the use of the time of our most senior clinicians and experienced supervisors but also exposing trainees to a broader array of patients and clinical situations than they might otherwise encounter in their own clinical practice.

FLEXIBLE IMPLEMENTATION

Mindful of research and training needs, we have attempted to present our approach to dynamic psychotherapy of higher level personality pathology in a fashion that is as clear, systematic, and detailed as possible. However, the clinical setting does not call for strictly adhering to a particular theory or technique. In fact, we have found that the most effective clinicians are typically those who consistently implement a particular psychotherapeutic approach, but in a fashion that is flexible rather than rigid and allows for some degree of deviation from standard technique to accommodate the particular clinical needs of each patient. Transient deviations from standard technique are to be expected, or one runs the risk of providing a perfectly adherent treatment that is ineffective because it fails to respond adequately to the individual patient. (We might say that this treatment is delivered in an adherent but not necessarily competent fashion.)

The need for flexible implementation is one reason we have chosen to emphasize *principles* of psychotherapeutic technique, especially strategies and tactics of treatment, rather than specific interventions. Our goal is not to leave the reader with an imperative to adhere rigidly to the psychotherapeutic technique described in this handbook. Rather, our hope is to leave the reader with a coherent way of thinking about dynamic psychotherapy. If we have done our job well, we have provided the reader with a systematic conceptual framework that he can turn to when reflecting on how to facilitate clinical process at any given moment or how to optimize therapeutic benefit in the long term. In sum, we hope that as clinicians of all experience levels come to understand and make use of the general principles and technical strategies in this handbook, they will develop their own personal version of the treatment we describe.

SUGGESTED READINGS

Caligor E: Treatment manuals for long-term psychodynamic psychotherapy and psychoanalysis. Clinical Neuroscience Research 4:387–398, 2005

Carroll KM, Nuro KF: One size cannot fit all: a stage model for psychotherapy manual development. Clinical Psychology: Science and Practice 9:396–406, 2002

REFERENCES

Akhtar S: Broken Structures: Severe Personality Disorders and Their Treatment. Northvale, NJ, Jason Aronson, 1992

American Psychiatric Association: Diagnostic and Statistical Manual of Mental Disorders, 4th Edition, Text Revision. Washington, DC, American Psychiatric Association, 2000

Apfelbaum B: Interpretive neutrality. J Am Psychoanal Assoc 53:917–943, 2005

Bateman A, Fonagy P: Psychotherapy for Borderline Personality: Mentalization-Based Treatment. New York, Oxford University Press, 2004

Beahrs JO, Gutheil TG: Informed consent in psychotherapy. Am J Psychiatry 158:4–10, 2001

Beck AH, Rush AJ, Shaw BF, et al: Cognitive Therapy of Depression. New York, Guilford, 1979

Bender DS: Therapeutic alliance, in The American Psychiatric Publishing Textbook of Personality Disorders. Edited by Oldham JM, Skodol AE, Bender DS. Washington, DC, American Psychiatric Publishing, 2005, pp 405–420

Beutler LE, Clarkin JF, Bongar B: Guidelines for the Systematic Treatment of the Depressed Patient. New York, Oxford, 2000

Bion WR: Attacks on linking (1959), in Second Thoughts. London, England, Heinemann, 1967, pp 93–109

Bion WR: Learning from Experience. London, England, Heinemann, 1962a

Bion WR: A theory of thinking (1962b), in Second Thoughts. London, England, Heinemann, 1967, pp 110–119

Bion WR: Elements of Psycho-Analysis. London, England, Heinemann, 1963

Bion WR: Notes on memory and desire. Psychoanalytic Forum 2:271–280, 1967a

Bion WR: Second Thoughts. Northvale, NJ, Jason Aronson, 1967b

Bretherton I: Internal working models: cognitive and affective aspects of attachment representations, in 4th Rochester Symposium on Developmental Psychopathology on "Emotion, Cognition, and Representation." Edited by Cichetti D, Toth S. Hillsdale, NJ, Erlbaum, 1995, pp 231–260

Britton R: Naming and containing, in Belief and Imagination. London, England, Routledge, 1998, pp 19–28

Busch F: The Ego at the Center of Clinical Technique. Northvale, NJ, Jason Aronson, 1995, pp 49–70

Busch F: The ego and its significance in analytic interventions. J Am Psychoanal Assoc 44:1073–1099, 1996

Caligor E: Treatment manuals for long-term psychodynamic psychotherapy and psychoanalysis. Clinical Neuroscience Research 4:387–398, 2005

Clark DA, Beck AT, Alford BA: Scientific Foundations of Cognitive Theory and Therapy of Depression. New York, John Wiley and Sons, 1999

Clarkin JF, Yeomans F, Kernberg OF: Psychotherapy for Borderline Personality: Focusing on Object Relations. Washington, DC, American Psychiatric Publishing, 2006

Costa P, Widiger TA: Personality Disorders and the Five-Factor Model of Personality. Washington, DC, American Psychiatric Publishing, 1994

Dubovsky SL, Davies R, Dubovsky AN: Mood disorders, in American Psychiatric Publishing Textbook of Clinical Psychiatry. Edited by Hales RE, Yudofsky SC. Washington, DC, American Psychiatric Publishing, 2003, pp 439–542

Erikson EH: The problem of ego identity, in Identity and the Life Cycle. New York, International Universities Press, 1956, pp 101–164

Etchegoyen RH: Fundamentals of Psychoanalytic Technique. London, England, Karnac Books, 1991

Fairbairn R: The repression and the return of bad objects (with special reference to the "War Neuroses") (1943), in Psychoanalytic Studies of Personality. London, England, Routledge, 1952, pp 59–81

Fenichel O: Problems of Psychoanalytic Technique. New York, Psychoanalytic Quarterly, 1941

Fonagy P: Attachment Theory and Psychoanalysis. New York, Other Press, 2001

Fonagy P, Target M: Psychoanalytic Theories: Perspectives from Developmental Psychopathology. London, England, Whurr Publishers, 2003, pp 270–282

Freud S: The interpretation of dreams (1900), in The Standard Edition of the Complete Psychological Works of Sigmund Freud, Vols 4–5. Edited and translated by Strachey J. London, Hogarth Press, 1953

Freud S: Inhibitions, symptoms and anxiety (1926), in The Standard Edition of the Complete Psychological Works of Sigmund Freud, Vol 20. Edited and translated by Strachey J. London, Hogarth Press, 1959, pp 77–175

Freud A: The ego and the mechanisms of defense (1937), in The Writings of Anna Freud, Vol II. New York, International Universities Press, 1966

Freud S: Letters to Wilhelm Fleiss, 1887–1902. New York, Basic Books, 1954

Gabbard GO: What can neuroscience teach us about transference? Canadian Journal of Psychoanalysis 9:1–18, 2001

Gabbard GO: Long-Term Psychodynamic Psychotherapy: A Basic Text. Washington, DC, American Psychiatric Publishing, 2004

Gabbard GO, Westen D: Rethinking therapeutic action. Int J Psychoanal 84:823–841, 2003

Gibbons MCG, Crits-Christoph P, de la Cruz C, et al: Pretreatment expectations, interpersonal functioning, and symptoms in the prediction of the therapeutic alliance across supportive-expressive psychotherapy and cognitive therapy. Psychother Res 13:59–76, 2003

Gutheil TG, Havens LL: The therapeutic alliance: contemporary meanings and confusions. International Review of Psychoanalysis 6:447–481, 1979

Harris A: Transference, countertransference and the real relationship, in The American Psychiatric Publishing Textbook of Psychoanalysis. Edited by Person ES, Cooper AM, Gabbard GO. Washington, DC, American Psychiatric Publishing, 2005, pp 201–216

Hinshelwood RD: A Dictionary of Kleinian Thought. Northvale, NJ, Jason Aronson, 1991

Hollander E, Simeon D: Anxiety Disorders, in The American Psychiatric Publishing Textbook of Clinical Psychiatry. Washington, DC, American Psychiatric Publishing, 2003, pp 543–631

Horvath AO, Greenberg LS (eds): The Working Alliance: Theory, Research and Practice. New York, Wiley, 1994

Horvath L, Symonds BD: Relation between working alliance and outcome in psychotherapy: a meta-analysis. J Couns Psychol 38:139–149, 1991

Joseph B: Projective identification, some clinical aspects (1987), in Melanie Klein Today, Vol. 1. Edited by Spillius EB. London, England, Routledge, 1988, pp 138–150

Kendler K, Kuhn J, Prescott CA: The interrelationship of neuroticism, sex, and stressful life events in the prediction of episodes of major depression. Am J Psychiatry 161:631–636, 2004

Kernberg OF: Countertransference, in Borderline Conditions and Pathological Narcissism. New York, Jason Aronson, 1975, pp 49–68

Kernberg OF: Object Relations Theory and Clinical Psychoanalysis. New York, Jason Aronson, 1976

Kernberg OF: Internal World and External Reality: Object Relations Theory Applied. New York, Jason Aronson, 1980

Kernberg OF: Severe Personality Disorders: Psychotherapeutic Strategies. New Haven, CT, Yale University Press, 1984

Kernberg OF: Aggression in Personality Disorders and Perversions. New Haven, CT, Yale University Press, 1992

Kernberg OF: Aggressivity, Narcissism, and Self-Destructiveness in the Psychotherapeutic Relationship. New Haven, CT, Yale University Press, 2004a

Kernberg OF: Contemporary Controversies in Psychoanalytic Theory, Techniques, and Their Applications. New Haven, CT, Yale University Press, 2004b

Kernberg OF: Identity: recent findings and clinical implications. Psychoanal Q 65:969–1004, 2006

Kernberg OF, Caligor E: A psychoanalytic theory of personality disorders, in Major Theories of Personality Disorder, 2nd Edition. Edited by Lenzenweger M, Clarkin JF. New York, Guilford, 2005, pp 114–156

Klein M: A contribution to the psychogenesis of manic-depressive states (1935), in Love, Guilt and Reparation and Other Works 1921–1945. London, England, Hogarth, 1975, pp 262–289

Klein M: Notes on some schizoid mechanisms (1946), in Envy and Gratitude and Other Works 1946–1963. New York, Free Press, 1975, pp 1–24

Klein M: Some theoretical conclusions regarding the emotional life of the infant (1952), in Envy and Gratitude and Other Works 1946–1963. New York, Free Press, 1975, pp 61–93

LaFarge L: Interpretation and containment. Int J Psychoanal 81:67–84, 2000

Lambert MJ, Ogles BM: The efficacy and effectiveness of psychotherapy, in Bergin and Garfield's Handbook of Psychotherapy and Behavior Change, 5th Edition. Edited by Lambert MJ. New York, Wiley, 2004, pp 139–193

Leichsenring F: Comparative effects of short-term psychodynamic psychotherapy and cognitive-behavioral therapy in depression: a meta-analytic approach. Clin Psychol Rev 21:401–419, 2001

Lenzenweger M, Clarkin J (eds): Major Theories of Personality Disorder, 2nd Edition. New York, Guilford, 2005

Lenzenweger MF, Clarkin, JK, Kernberg OF, et al: The Inventory of Personality Organization: psychometric properties, factorial composition and criterion relations with affects, aggressive dyscontrol, psychosis-proneness, and self domains. Psychol Assess 4:577–591, 2001

Levy KN, Kelly KM, Meehan KB, et al: Change in attachment patterns and reflective function in a randomized control trial of transference focused psychotherapy for borderline personality disorder. J Consult Clin Psychol 62:481–501, 2006

Levy ST, Inderbitzin LB: Neutrality, interpretation and therapeutic intent. J Am Psychoanal Assoc 40:989–1011, 1992

Loewald H: On the therapeutic action of psychoanalysis. Int J Psychoanal 41:16–33, 1960

Luborsky L: Principles of Psychoanalytic Psychotherapy: A Manual for Supportive-Expressive Treatment. New York, Basic Books, 1984

Luborsky L, DeRubeis R: The use of psychotherapy manuals: a small revolution in psychotherapy research style. Clin Psychol Rev 4:5–14, 1984

Malan D: Individual Psychotherapy and the Science of Psychodynamics, 2nd Edition. New York, Oxford University Press, 2004

Marmar CR, Horowitz MJ, Weiss DS, et al: The development of the therapeutic alliance rating system, in The Psychotherapeutic Process. Edited by Greenberg LS, Pinsof WM. New York, Guilford, 1986, pp 367–390

McWilliams N: Narcissistic personalities, in Psychoanalytic Diagnosis: Understanding Personality Structure in the Clinical Process. New York, Guilford, 1994, pp 168–188

Moore BE, Fine D: Psychoanalysis: The Major Concepts. New Haven, CT, Yale University Press, 1995

Ogden TH: Projective Identification and Psychotherapeutic Technique (1982). Northvale, NJ, Jason Aronson, 1993

Oldham JM, Skodol AF: Charting the future of Axis II. J Personal Disord 14:30–41, 2000

Orlinsky DE, Ronnestad MH, Willutzki U: Fifty years of psychotherapy process-outcome research: continuity and change, in Bergin and Garfield's Handbook of Psychotherapy and Behavior Change, 5th Edition. Edited by Lambert MJ. New York, Wiley, 1994, pp 307–390

PDM Task Force: Psychodynamic Diagnostic Manual, Personality Patterns and Disorders. Silver Spring, MD, Alliance of Psychoanalytic Organizations, 2006

Perry JC, Bond M: Defensive functioning, in The American Psychiatric Publishing Textbook of Personality Disorders. Edited by Oldham JM, Skodol AE, Bender DS. Washington, DC, American Psychiatric Publishing, 2005, pp 523–540

Piper WE, Duncan SC: Object relations theory and short-term dynamic psychotherapy: findings from the quality of object relations scale. Clin Psychol Rev 19:669–685, 1999

Piper WE, Azim HFA, Joyce AS, et al: Quality of object relations versus interpersonal functioning as predictors of therapeutic alliance and psychotherapy outcome. J Nerv Ment Dis 179:432–438, 1991

Racker H: The meaning and uses of countertransference. Psychoanal Q 26:303–357, 1957

Rangell L: The self in psychoanalytic theory. J Am Psychoanal Assoc 30:863–891, 1982

Rockland L: Supportive Therapy: A Psychodynamic Approach. New York, Basic Books, 1989

Rush AJ, Trivedi MH, Wisniewski SR, et al: Acute and longer-term outcomes in depressed outpatients requiring one or several treatment steps: a STAR*D report. Am J Psychiatry 163:1905–1917, 2006

Sandell R, Blomberg J, Lazar A, et al: Varieties of long-term outcome among patients in psychoanalysis and long-term psychotherapy: a review of findings in the Stockholm Outcome of Psychoanalysis and Psychotherapy Project (STOPP). Int J Psychoanal 81:921–943, 2000

Sandler J: The background of safety. Paper presented at the 21st Congress of the International Psychoanalytical Association, Copenhagen, Denmark, July 1959

Sandler J: Countertransference and role responsiveness. International Review of Psychoanalysis 3:43–47, 1976

Sandler J: From Safety to Superego: Selected Papers of Joseph Sandler. New York, Guilford Press, 1987

Sandler J: On attachment to internal objects. Psychoanalytic Inquiry 23:12–26, 2003

Sandler J, Dare C, Holder H: The Patient and the Analyst, 2nd Edition. Madison, CT, International Universities Press, 1992

Schafer R: The Analytic Attitude. New York, Basic Books, 1983

Schafer R: The interpretation of psychic reality, developmental influences, and unconscious communication. J Am Psychoanal Assoc 33:537–554, 1985

Schlesinger HJ: Endings and Beginnings: On Terminating Psychotherapy and Psychoanalysis. Hillsdale, NJ, Analytic Press, 2005

Segal H: An Introduction to the Work of Melanie Klein. New York, Basic Books, 1964

Skodol AE, Oldham JM, Bender DS, et al: Dimensional representations of DSM-IV personality disorders: relationship to functional impairment. Am J Psychiatry 162:1919–1926, 2005

Smith HF: Analysis of transference: a North American perspective. Int J Psychoanal 84:1017–1041, 2003

Spillius EB: Development in Kleinian thought: overview and personal view. Psychoanalytic Inquiry 14:324–364, 1994

Steiner J: The equilibrium between the paranoid-schizoid and the depressive positions, in Clinical Lectures on Klein and Bion. London, England, Routledge, 1992, pp 34–45

Steiner J: Psychic Retreats. London, England, Routledge, 1993

Steiner J: Patient-centered and analyst-centered interpretations. Psychoanalytic Inquiry 14:406–422, 1994

Steiner J: The aim of psychoanalysis in theory and practice. Int J Psychoanal 77:1073–1083, 1996

Steiner J: Interpretive enactments and the analytic setting. Int J Psychoanal 87:315–320, 2006

Sullivan HS: The Psychiatric Interview. New York, WW Norton, 1970, p 3

Thase ME, Entsuah AR, Rudolph RL: Remission rates during treatment with venlafaxine or selective serotonin reuptake inhibitors. Br J Psychiatry 178:234–241, 2001

Vaillant G: Ego Mechanisms of Defense: A Guide for Clinicians and Researchers. Washington DC, American Psychiatric Press, 1992

Vaillant G: The Wisdom of the Ego. Cambridge, MA, Harvard University Press, 1993

Westen D, Arkowitz-Westen L: Limitations of Axis II in diagnosing personality pathology in clinical practice. Am J Psychiatry 155:1767–1771, 1998

Westen D, Gabbard G: Developments in cognitive neuroscience, II: implications for theories of transference. J Am Psychoanal Assoc 50:99–134, 2002

Westen D, Schedler J: Revising and assessing Axis II, part I: developing a clinically and empirically valid assessment method. Am J Psychiatry 156:258–272, 1999a

Westen D, Schedler J: Revising and assessing Axis II, part II: toward an empirically based and clinically useful classification of personality disorders. Am J Psychiatry 156:273–285, 1999b

Widiger TA: The DSM-III-R categorical personality disorders diagnoses: a critique and an alternative. Psychological Inquiry 4:75–90, 1993

Widiger TA, Mullins-Sweatt SN: Categorical and dimensional models of personality disorders, in The American Psychiatric Publishing Textbook of Personality Disorders. Edited by Oldham JM, Skodol AE, Bender DS. Washington, DC, American Psychiatric Publishing, 2005, pp 35–56

INDEX

Page numbers printed in **boldface** *type refer to figures or tables.*